# Metaphors of Mental Illness in Graphic Medicine

This book investigates how graphic medicine enables sufferers of mental illness to visualise the intricacies of their internal mindscape through visual metaphors and reclaim their voice amidst stereotyped and prejudiced assumptions of mental illness as a disease of deviance and violence.

In this context, by using Lakoff and Johnson's conceptual metaphor theory (CMT), this study uncovers the broad spectrum of the mentally ills' experiences, a relatively undertheorised area in medical humanities. The aim is to demonstrate that mentally ill people are often represented as either grotesquely exaggerated or overly romanticised across diverse media and biomedical discourses. Further, they have been disparaged as emotionally drained and unreasonable individuals, incapable of active social engagements and against the healthy/sane society.

The study also aims to unsettle the sanity/insanity binary and its related patterns of fixed categories of normal/abnormal, which depersonalise the mentally ill by critically analysing seven graphic narratives on mental illness.

**Sweetha Saji** is Assistant Professor in the Department of English at Mount Carmel College, Bengaluru. Her areas of research interest include Graphic Medicine and Medical Humanities. She has published over ten research articles in SCI and Scopus indexed journals. She is an ad-hoc reviewer for *Journal of Graphic Novels and Comics* and *BMJ Journal of Medical Humanities.* She has presented over 12 research papers at International and National conferences organized by prestigious institutions including the University of Granada, Spain, JNU New Delhi, and IIT Madras.

**Sathyaraj Venkatesan** is Associate Professor of English in the Department of Humanities and Social Sciences at the National Institute of Technology, Trichy (India). He is the author of 6 books and over 90 research publications that span African American literature, health humanities, graphic medicine, film studies, and other literary and culture studies disciplines. He is most recently the co-author of *Infertility Comics and Graphic Medicine* (2021) and *India Retold* (2021).

# Routledge Focus on Literature

**Trump and Autobiography**
Corporate Culture, Political Rhetoric, and Interpretation
*Nicholas K. Mohlmann*

**Biofictions**
Literary and Visual Imagination in the Age of Biotechnology
*Lejla Kucukalic*

**Neurocognitive Interpretations of Australian Literature**
Criticism in the Age of Neuroawareness
*Jean-François Vernay*

**Mapping the Origins of Figurative Language in Comparative Literature**
*Richard Trim*

**Metaphors of Mental Illness in Graphic Medicine**
*Sweetha Saji and Sathyaraj Venkatesan*

**Wanderers**
Literature, Culture and the Open Road
*David Brown Morris*

**Sham Ruins**
A User's Guide
*Brian Willems*

For more information about this series, please visit: www.routledge.com/Routledge-Focus-on-Literature/book-series/RFLT

# Metaphors of Mental Illness in Graphic Medicine

Sweetha Saji and
Sathyaraj Venkatesan

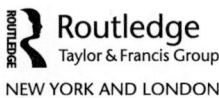

Routledge
Taylor & Francis Group

NEW YORK AND LONDON

First published 2022
by Routledge
605 Third Avenue, New York, NY 10158

and by Routledge
2 Park Square, Milton Park, Abingdon, Oxon, OX14 4RN

*Routledge is an imprint of the Taylor & Francis Group, an informa business*

*Library of Congress Cataloging-in-Publication Data*
Names: Saji, Sweetha, author. | Venkatesan, Sathyaraj, author.
Title: Metaphors of mental illness in graphic medicine / Sweetha Saji, Sathyaraj Venkatesan.
Description: New York, NY : Routledge, 2022. | Series: Routledge focus on literature | Includes bibliographical references and index.
Identifiers: LCCN 2021032613
Subjects: LCSH: Mental illness—Treatment. | Visualization.
Classification: LCC RC475 .S25 2022 | DDC 616.891—dc23
LC record available at https://lccn.loc.gov/2021032613

ISBN: 9781032102092 (hbk)
ISBN: 9781032163505 (pbk)
ISBN: 9781003214229 (ebk)

DOI: 10.4324/9781003214229

Typeset in Times New Roman
by codeMantra

# Contents

# Acknowledgements

I am grateful to Dr Sathyaraj Venkatesan, who has taught me the art of academic writing and guided me throughout the course of four years as a researcher. My gratitude also extends to my teachers of SB College, Changanacherry, and BCM College, Kottayam, for inspiring me to develop academic curiosity which led me to venture into the novel interdisciplinary fields of medical humanities and graphic medicine.

Immense thanks to Brick, Rachel Lindsay, Nate Powell, and Glyn Dillon who spared their precious time in sending me images from their memoirs. I fondly remember William Kuskin of the University of Colorado Boulder and Andrea Wood of Winona State University for their insightful comments and valuable suggestions on this book. I am grateful to Matthew Noe of Harvard Medical School for his specific comments on this book and also for the effort he takes to compile all the resources related to this new field of graphic medicine and sharing the same with the graphic medicine community online.

I am thankful to Jennifer Abbot, Mitchell Manners, and all the editorial and production team members at Routledge, New York, and Rajamalar of CodeMantra for their timely suggestions and help during the various stages of the production of this book. I thankfully remember the support given by the librarians at the American Corner; Kottayam Public Library; Jawaharlal Nehru University, New Delhi; Indian Institute of Technology, Madras; and National Institute of Technology, Trichy.

My sincere gratitude and respect to my parents and siblings for their encouragement and prayers. My heartfelt love and thanks to my husband, Gijo John George, for his unconditional support. Special thanks to S. Pushpanathan, Rajima, Ninu, and Geerthy for their unflinching friendship and love.

I thank the publishers of Routledge, Sage, Rupkatha, and Media Watch, for permitting me to use earlier versions of some of the chapters in this book which were published as "Drawing the Mind: Aesthetics of Representing Mental Illness in Select Graphic Memoirs" in *Health: An International Journal for Social Study of Health, Illness and Medicine*, Sage vol. 25, no.1 (2021); "Capturing Alternate Realities: Visual Metaphors and Patient Perspectives in Graphic Narratives on Mental Illness" in *Journal of Graphic Novels and Comics* (2020); "Reflections on the Visceral: Metaphors and Illness Experience" in *Rupkatha Journal on Interdisciplinary Studies in Humanities* vol.12, no.1 (2020); "Graphic Illness Memoirs as Counter-Discourse" in *Journal of Graphic Novels and Comics* (2019); and "Conjuring the 'Insane': Representations of Mental Illness in Medical and Popular Discourses" in *Media Watch* vol.10, no.3 (2019).

This book is dedicated to my family and all my teachers who moulded me through these years. They seeded in me empathy, the foundation on which this book is thought about and made.

Sweetha Saji

My special debt of gratitude to Professor Gurumurthy Neelakantan, Indian Institute of Technology, Kanpur, for teaching me the art of interpretation and academic writing. I would like to thank Jennifer Abbott and Mitchell Manners for their utmost professionalism and enthusiasm during the preparation of the manuscript. My deep sense of gratitude to the International Graphic Medicine collective for their extraordinary support: Dr Ian Williams (founder of Graphic Medicine), MK Czerwiec (co-founder of Graphic Medicine), Susan Merrill Squier, Dr Michael Green (Penn State College of Medicine), Matthew Noe (Harvard Medical School), A David Lewis (Massachusetts College of Pharmacy and Health Sciences), Dr Brian Callender (University of Chicago), and Larry Churchill (University of Vanderbilt). Thanks to the reviewers for their thoughtful critiques and valuable suggestions. Thanks to William Kuskin (University of Colorado, Boulder) for being a great source of motivation. Special thanks are due to the faculty of the Department of Humanities and Social Sciences, National Institute of Technology (NIT), Tiruchirappalli. Thanks also to the publishers who allowed to reproduce essays contained in this book. Dedicated to my wife, Pavithra Ayyapan, and my son, Taran Sathyaraj.

Sathyaraj Venkatesan

# Introduction

'

The pivotal role of humanities in medicine has been recognised in the 1940s as it aimed at reuniting technical and humanistic theory and practice. Since then, discussions on the interdisciplinary field of health humanities promoted the inculcation of humane values and concerns within medical practice by exposing students of medicine to literature, culture, philosophy, and the arts. Steering away from symptom-based approaches, health humanities foreground patient-centred care that takes into account varied socio-cultural factors that modulate and determine one's experience of illness. Moreover, the field shies away from privileging singular perspectives and grants voice to the care provider as well as to the patient. Broadening the scope of this field, later developments in health humanities like narrative medicine among others explore questions of empathy, narrative humility, and ethics of representation. Taking cues from these historical milestones, the field of graphic medicine, which explores representations of illness experiences in the medium of comics, "resists the notion of the universal patient and vividly represents multiple subjects with valid and, at times, conflicting points of view and experiences" (Czerwiec et al. 2). Within this framework, the experience of mental illness becomes significant as it is often misrepresented in various verbal, visual, and media cultures. Such representations promote stereotypes and affect the very social and personal well-being of the mentally ill. In this context, personal narratives of mental illness experience grant agency to such marginal lives and thus provide an alternate perspective to the current (toxic) discourses on mental illness.

As such, the COVID-19 pandemic has reanimated several issues about mental health and well-being. Quarantine, isolation, and social distancing which are the recommended measures to limit the spread of the viral disease have not only resulted in socio-cultural and economic crisis but also have led to personal disruption and extreme

DOI: 10.4324/9781003214229-1

mental health issues. As a response, health professionals discuss the importance of attending to the needs of the mentally ill and being sensitive to those who suffer mental health issues during the pandemic. Artists and writers, on the other hand, have creatively engaged in such invisible dimensions of one's life and also have elicited (empathetic) responses via print and social media. Such emerging trends not only extend ingress into the subjective dimensions of patient experience but also bring under scrutiny the extant medical practices and popular representations of madness that underrepresent or over romanticise the experience of mental illness. Graphic memoirs on mental illness, in particular, find expression through the unique semiotic nature of comics, which facilitates the encapsulation of complex psychic landscapes and embodiment of the artist's experiences. Such representations of psychological experiences that concern with challenging prevailing normativities necessitate a creative use of means of expression. In so doing, these verbo-visual techniques such as the use of visual metaphors provide vividness and easily digested expression, translating the sufferer's altered mental perspective effectively for the reader. The deployment of such elements inherent in the medium facilitates multi-layered connections to the patient narrative which provide a depth beyond the raw medical discourse, and thereby reconfigures the extant perceptions surrounding mental illness.

An analysis of diverse verbal and visual representations of mental illness in contemporary media and medical discourses reveals a persistent gap between standardised and stereotyped perspectives about the mentally ill and the subjective realisation of them. Several literary and cultural critics have commented on this glaring lacunae and its negative repercussions on the personal, familial, and social life of the mentally ill. Sander Gilman's *Seeing the Insane* (1982), Simon Cross' *Mediating Madness: Mental Distress and Cultural Representation* (2010), and Elizabeth J. Donaldson's *Literatures of Madness: Disability Studies and Mental Health* (2018) are some of the seminal critical readings on representations of the mentally ill across media and its unconstructive effects. While these texts explore the politics of representation and its repercussions in the lives of the mentally ill, a critical reading of personal narratives of mental illness which are drafted using verbal and visual modes unravels the unvoiced socio-cultural and personal dimensions of living with mental illness from significant marginal perspectives. As such, a nuanced understanding of the affordances of the comics medium and the metaphorical patterns which recur in these graphic narratives enables a comprehensive reading experience which generates a community of sufferers on the one hand and facilitates critical responses on health and illness on the other hand.

Although concepts and theories on metaphors date back to Aristotle, current research on metaphors, particularly visual metaphors, draws strength from George Lakoff and Mark Johnson's conceptual metaphor theory (CMT) which deems metaphors to be "pervasive in everyday life, not just in language but in thought and action" (3). Lakoff and Johnson and other theorists like Charles Forceville and Elizabeth El Refaie primarily focus on the cognitive mapping between two different conceptual categories that evoke metaphorical meanings that arise "from the continuous interplay of social and cultural constraints, neural processing, and the unfolding of in-the-moment sensorimotor experience" (El Refaie 4). These meanings that emerge out of such conceptual mappings actualise otherwise abstract feelings and emotions that require a visual language that transcends literal expressions. In the context of mental illness, the author/artist resorts to metaphors which effectively encapsulate their complex psychic landscapes which seldom find expression in literal language due to the absence of physical/visible signs of illness. Although Lakoff and Johnson's CMT is extended to visual narratives to investigate "the correspondence between the *visual* form and meaning" (Cohn 68), artists also deploy metonymic relationships between images and "unseen events" (Cohn 80). In other words, when graphic narratives use metaphor, it is usually through another aspect of metonymy—polysemy—in which something is figured in multiple ways, through visualisation and through text. As such, in a visual medium like comics, artists use panels to "show something related to an event, without showing the event itself" (Cohn 80). These 'unseen events' correspond to what Ian Williams defines as the 'invisible' iconography used in depicting psychological conditions (Czerwiec et al. 119).

Under the rubrics of the iconography of illness in the medium of comics, Williams classifies illness representation into 'the manifest,' 'the concealed,' and 'the invisible.' 'The manifest' implies the depiction of illness or scars of treatment "as 'realistically' as possible" (Czerwiec et al. 121). Drawing specific attention to David Small's memoir, *Stitches*, Williams enunciates the usefulness of 'manifest' images in rendering physical/bodily scars. Such graphic depiction which converges sickness with grotesqueness consequently evokes disgust/pity in the reader. When illness conditions are vaguely manifest as in the case of psychosomatic disorders, Williams christens it as 'the concealed.' In such cases, Williams remarks that they "may not be noticed by, or are hidden from, the casual observer" (Czerwiec et al. 119). In the third category of illness depiction called 'the invisible,' the comic artist resorts to the "iconographic flexibility of the form" (Czerwiec et al. 119) for the veracious articulation of the visceral and analytic dimensions of psychological suffering. Exploiting the flexibility of the comics medium, the artists choose/create idiosyncratic icons and experiment with visual tropes creating new visual patterns and an internal vocabulary of images to align with their peculiarity of experience. Several mental illness graphic narratives such as Ellen Forney's *Marbles*, Allie Brosh's *Hyperbole and a Half*, Darryl Cunnigham's *Psychiatric Tales*, Elaine Will's *Look Straight Ahead*, and Steven Struble's *Li'l Depressed Boy,* among others, exploit the iconographic flexibility of the comics medium in order to concretise and effectively relate their mental states through visual metaphors.

## Texts and Contexts

This book critically analyses seven graphic narratives on mental illness, namely, Nate Powell's *Swallow Me Whole* (2008), Brick's *Depresso* (2010), Darryl Cunnigham's *Psychiatric Tales* (2011), Ellen Forney's *Marbles* (2012), Glyn Dillon's *The Nao of Brown* (2012), Allie Brosh's *Hyperbole and a Half* (2013), and Rachel Lindsay's *Rx* (2018). These narratives include both fictional and non-fictional accounts that deal with mental illnesses including bipolar disorder, depression, schizophrenia, and obsessive compulsive disorder (OCD). The primary texts were selected on the basis of their delineation of experiential dimension of the sufferer's life, and their use of comics as a medium of expression in exploring cultural and emotional aspects of the illness through different kinds of metaphors that convey their unique emotional landscapes. The authors comprise established comic artists and blog writers who suffer(ed) from various forms of mental illness. The study also aims to inspire qualitative and quantitative research on how factors such as gender, ethnicity, and race influence and determine (mental) illness conditions.

First, we follow a phenomenological approach which aims to capture the lived realities of those who suffer from mental illness. This approach respects the perspective of those affected by the illness condition by being aware of the personal, socio-cultural, and paradigmatic discourses that shape the way reality is perceived by them. Second, the core chapters specifically follow certain tenets of poststructuralism that problematise social and medical discourses on mental illness that mediate the way in which the illness condition and sufferers of the same are perceived. Accordingly, the binaries that underpin negative attitudes towards mental illness are deconstructed through concepts like counter-space and counter-diagnosis. Analysis of visual and verbo-visual metaphors in the graphic memoirs which are close-read in this book reveals how the authors subvert institu-tionalised structures of power through creative ways that foreground subjective dimensions of living with mental illness. Third, by follow-ing a contextualist methodological approach, few primary texts are close-read based on its socio-cultural contexts and its connections to the lived body experience of those suffering from mental illnesses like OCD and schizophrenia. These approaches problematise monolithic and singular notions of 'truth' as available in biomedical/diagnostic discourses and lay bare multiple perspectives and realities of an illness experience.

The term 'madness' would be used in this book as a cultural marker; a "generic name for the whole range of people thought to be in some way, more or less, abnormal in ideas or behaviour" (Porter 6). The term 'mental illness' would be used to refer to the experiential aspects of living with mental conditions that influence one's emotions and behaviour. The fourth chapter initiates an investigation of such con-tradictory and ambivalent notions about the mentally ill that contrib-ute to their stigma and examines the obstructions that hinder a lucid understanding of the experiential dimensions of living with mental illness.

As the subtitles of several autobiographical comics evince, there is a persistent anxiety about the generic classification of such narra-tives. For instance, subtitles such as 'a comic-strip narrative' (Chester Brown's *I Never Like You* [1994]), 'graphic stories' (Darryl Cunning-ham's *Psychiatric Tales* [2010]), and 'graphic memoir' (Rachel Lind-say's *Rx* [2018]) challenge a standard definition of the form of these narratives on mental illness. Although a wide range of terms (such as comics, graphic novels, and graphic narratives, apart from the ones mentioned above) are used to refer to verbo-visual narratives, the term 'comics' is used as a singular noun in this book to refer to the medium. As Hillary Chute defines, comics is "a hybrid word-and-image form in which two narrative tracks, one verbal and one visual, register tempo-rality spatially" (452). While 'graphic narratives' is used as a broader term to refer to a "book-length work in the medium of comics" (Chute 453), the term 'graphic memoir' is used in this book to refer specifically to personal accounts in the medium of comics about a particular phase of life (here, the experience of living with mental illness). Fictional ac-counts of mental illness in this book are referred to as 'graphic novels.'

The graphic narratives discussed in this book use both images and words where the text accompanying the image "adds some unillus-trated thoughts hand-lettered in a style that is consistent with the sen-timent that its message conveys" (Eisner 10). As Francisca Goldsmith observes, "image and text are [typically] brought together within panels or defined spaces on the page, but in some instances the entire page may serve as a panel" (4). The close-readings of particular episodes are based on the theoretical findings of Scott McCloud and Thierry Groensteen. While McCloud's sequential reading of panels enables a detailed understanding of the diverse comic elements that the authors deploy within each panel to evoke specific meanings, Groensteen's principles of "arthrology" (linear relation of panels to each other) and "braiding" (connection across the multiframe of the comics page) enable a broader understanding of the comics page as a whole in translating the mental landscape of the characters (Beaty and Nguyen).

## Overview of the Book

This book consists of six core chapters and a conclusion, and each chapter is followed by a reference list. This introductory chapter has aimed at providing a brief outline of the objectives, scope and the methodology of the study.

Chapter 1, "Drawing Illness: History, Theory, and the Development of Graphic Medicine," charts the development of graphic medicine by tracing the engagement of comics with healthcare across time. Subsequently, the chapter explores the role of comics in medical training; appraises seminal graphic pathographies on physical illness, mental illness, and disability; and discusses the significance of multiple perspectives on illness which provide a depth beyond monolithic biomedical approach toward patient bodies. As such, the chapter espouses the significance of graphic medicine in validating the affective truths about illness and health in treatment and recovery by underscoring the need to acknowledge the sufferer's voice. Apart from delineating the cultural role of graphic medicine, the chapter also clarifies the various elements of the comics medium which distinguishes graphic pathographies from educational health comics in terms of style, target audience, and production. The chapter further elaborates on the recent trends and global recognition of graphic medicine as an emerging interdisciplinary field.

Chapter 2, "Function of Metaphors in Illness Narratives," aims to provide a systematic reflection on metaphor as an expression of lived experience. The chapter will also provide an overview of the major theories on metaphors with an emphasis on Lakoff and Johnson's CMT since the implications of the theory correspond to the objectives of graphic medicine. Furthermore, the wider implications of using multimodal metaphors, especially visual and verbo-visual metaphors in graphic memoirs, will be analysed in the context of mental illness.

The chapter also elaborates on Susan Sontag's seminal work, *Illness as Metaphor*, and recent theoretical postulates regarding the use of metaphors in representing illness and its implications.

Drawing theoretical insights from Paula A. Treichler and Stuart Hall, Chapter 3, "Mental Illness and the Politics of Representation," analyses perceptions and representations of mental illness in popular culture and medical discourses. In so doing, the chapter lays bare the ideologies and the symbolic codes that undergird these representations in paintings, movies, television shows, advertisements, newspaper reports, and medical illustrations. Invoking the diverse definitions and perspectives on mental illness, the chapter also explores how stereotyped popular and medical representations of the marginalised, especially the mentally ill, engender internal and social stigma which impedes recovery and social life. In this context, the chapter emphasises the significance of personal accounts as a means to reconfigure popular perceptions that threaten the personal and social life of the mentally ill.

Negotiating the gaps and misconceptions that permeate the popular and biomedical discourses, Chapter 4, "Nobody Memoirs as Counter-Discourse: Bipolar Disorder and Its Metaphors," aims to explore the diverse ways in which memoirs on mental illness construct a counter-discourse by challenging and subverting the stereotypical representations of madness. Specifically, the chapter investigates the function of visual metaphors as a tool of counter-diagnosis which shape the characterisation of different embodiments in graphic memoirs. Moreover, the chapter investigates how these metaphors grant agency to the patients to control the representation of one's own illness. Drawing from Thomas Couser's concept of 'nobody memoirs,' the chapter facilitates the analysis of graphic memoirs on bipolar disorder like *Marbles* and *Rx* which explains how these artists deploy metaphors to question medical dogma on the one hand and the binaries of sanity and insanity on the other.

Chapter 5, "Visual Metaphors of OCD and Schizophrenia," close-reads graphic narratives on mental illnesses like schizophrenia and OCD, namely, *Swallow Me Whole* and *Nao of Brown* to argue that spatio-temporal affordance of the comics medium facilitates the representation of specific embodied states. In foregrounding patient perspectives, the chapter elaborates on spatial and stylistic metaphors that simulate uncontrollable and parallel thoughts that are characteristic of schizophrenia and OCD. Furthermore, the chapter analyses cultural confluences and identity crises of the protagonists through contextual metaphors which encourage readers to comprehend a concept in terms of another through replacement of anticipated contextual elements.

Chapter 6, "Visualising the Fragmented Selves: Conventional and Creative Metaphors of Depression," investigates the mediative value of conventional and creative metaphors unique to the medium of comics in actualising the subjective experience of mental illness. The chapter also seeks to delineate the cultural role of graphic memoirs by positioning them at the crossroads of sufferer's experiences and clinical description, drawing on theoretical insights from Lakoff and Johnson and other graphic pathographers/theorists, such as Williams and El Refaie. Focussing particularly on graphic memoirs on depression such as *Psychiatric Tales*, *Depresso*, and *Hyperbole and a Half*, the chapter explores the rhetoric of picturing the fragmented sense of self which is characteristic of depressed mental conditions. The chapter further discusses how creative metaphors and creative page layout are used in these memoirs to establish an authentic subjective voice that departs from the standards of symptomatic biomedical approach to illness and health.

The conclusion draws together the principal findings of the study and proposes new directions towards further research in the use of visual metaphors in graphic memoirs on mental illness experience. The limitations of the study are also discussed in the conclusion. In essence, we seek to expand the boundaries of interdisciplinary research on comics and healthcare with regard to mental illness.

## Reference List

Beaty, Bart, and Nick Nguyen, translators. *The System of Comics*. By Theirry Groensteen, UP of Mississippi, 2007.

Chute, Hillary. "Comics as Literature? Reading Graphic Narrative." *PMLA*, vol. 123, no. 2, 2008, pp. 452–465.

Cohn, Neil. "Being Explicit about the Implicit: Inference Generating Techniques in Visual Narrative." *Language and Cognition*, vol. 11, 2019, pp. 66–97.

Czerwiec, M. K., et al. *Graphic Medicine Manifesto*. The Pennsylvania State UP, 2015.

Eisner, Will. *Comics & Sequential Art*. Poorhouse, 1985.

El Refaie, Elisabeth. *Visual Metaphor and Embodiment in Graphic Illness Narratives*. Oxford UP, 2019.

Goldsmith, Francisca. *The Readers' Advisory Guide to Graphic Novels*. American Library Association, 2010.

Lakoff, George, and Mark Johnson. *Metaphors We Live By: With a New Afterword*. The U of Chicago P, 2003.

Porter, Roy. *A Social History of Madness*. Weidenfeld & Nicolson, 1987.

# 1  Drawing Illness

## History, Theory, and the Development of Graphic Medicine

### Introduction

Appraising comics within their constraints and possibilities, one could contend that their verbal, non-verbal, and para-linguistic attributes relay intimacy and inter-subjective experiences through a range of structural and formal properties. As such, a new genre of comics has emerged in the past decade that productively utilises this medium's immense potential to portray patients', caregivers', and healthcare professionals' illness experiences. This diverse and novel approach to arts and medicine has ushered in new modes to address subjective experiences of illness that transcend the prescribed boundaries of biomedicine and canonical literature. British doctor and graphic novelist Ian Williams labelled this approach to comics 'graphic medicine,' which is defined as "the intersection of the medium of comics and the discourse of health care" (Czerwiec et al. 1). These graphic illness narratives (also called graphic pathographies), which are mostly autobiographical, also address various socio-cultural issues impinging upon healthcare, such as the demands placed on doctors in a commercialised healthcare sector, medical negligence, the industrialisation of healthcare, the doctor-patient relationship, patient identity, and the challenges of patient care. Tracing the engagement of comics with healthcare across time, this chapter elucidates the development of graphic medicine. Subsequently, this chapter explores the role of comics in medical training; appraises seminal graphic pathographies on physical illness, mental illness, and disability; and discusses the significance of exposing multiple perspectives on illness and thus provides a depth beyond the monolithic biomedical approach toward patients.

DOI: 10.4324/9781003214229-2

## Early Comics and Healthcare

McCloud drew a comparison, saying that if comics could be defined as a narration of events using words and images, then its origins could be traced back to Egyptian hieroglyphics, Greek paintings, Japanese scrolls, and Bayeux tapestry, which belong between the seventh and twelfth centuries (12, 15). However, the beginning of modern comics is more often traced to the "picture stories" (Kunzle xi) of Rodolphe Töpffer, an early nineteenth-century Swiss schoolmaster. Töpffer established the new genre on broadsheets with multiple images on a single page (Kunzle 75). In horizontal albums, usually consisting of one tier with many panels, Töpffer created his stories, which were to be read linearly. However, in place of speech bubbles as found in later years, Patricia Mainardi explains that Töpffer handwrote his captions below each drawing (2). Although his narratives had no special effects, like zooming or layout distortions, he maintained the "boxed grid format with handwritten text below" (Mainardi 3). Inspired by Töpffer, artists like Cham and Gustave Doré adopted a similar sequential album style with improvised drawings and shading. Cham experimented with the style subsequently by eliminating boxed frames and handwritten captions and replaced them with typeface and arranged frames, spread freely across the page and which could be read in any direction. By contrast, Doré maintained Töpffer's style of drawing with the handwritten caption and panels that were to be read horizontally. However, according to Mainardi, Doré "exploited the rhythm of turning pages with the element of surprise" and invented the convention of "speed lines" (9). Notably, each of these early artists exploited the potential of the medium to comment on and satirise contemporary society.

The comics produced in later years also engaged with socio-cultural issues impinging upon healthcare. In his essay, "The Image and Advocacy of Public Health in American Caricature and Cartoons from 1860 to 1900," Bert Hansen argues that an examination of the popular cartoon images of public health enriches the "historical understanding of ordinary citizens' awareness of the public health issues," and explicates "how a large segment of the public 'saw' public health" (1798). Striving for change and advocacy, these cartoons, which were featured in magazines and newspapers of the late nineteenth century, "selected targets [and] uncovered less visible problems" concerning public nuisances, quarantine and immigration, and food purity and adulteration (1798). By influencing and altering public perceptions about politics and healthcare, cartoons by artists like Thomas Nast and Joseph Keppler served as vital tools that initiated social and cultural changes.

Newspapers like *Frank Leslie's Illustrated Newspaper* deliberately exploited the power of images and words to move people into action.

During the period of the 1930s to the 1950s, comics and medicine had a parallel rise in popularity, which historians refer to as the golden age of each of these disciplines. As such, emulating the ethos of the superhero cult, numerous healthcare and scientific themes found representation in the medium of comic strips. While the golden age of comics created a range of superheroes, comics grounded in medical history helped to reinforce the rising status of the American medical profession. As such, comic books like *True Comics, Real Heroes,* and *Real Life Comics* depicted real life heroes of the post-war era—Louis Pasteur, Florence Nightingale, Theobald Smith, and several others. As the trend in comics gradually shifted from superheroes to real-life stories, the primary motive in these also shifted from entertainment to information. In 1941, *True Comics* emerged as a definitive subgenre in comics, with the motto, according to Hansen, "TRUTH is stranger and a thousand times more thrilling than FICTION" ("Medical History" 159; emphasis in the original). As *True Comics* quickly became popular, with numerous sister publications like *Real Heroes* and *Real Life Comics,* Hansen argues that a significantly large readership was created for medical history among American teenagers (161). The healthcare professionals in these narratives were described and depicted as potential role models endowed with the value of heroism and as having quests for discoveries (162). Hinged on the climax of a remarkable medical breakthrough, most of these narratives catered to triumphalism (167). As a primarily informative genre aimed at instilling such values as hard work and virtue, these comics and hagiographies did not necessarily adhere to historical accuracy (168). Some of the prominent graphic hagiographies of the time include Gary Gray's "Louis Pasteur," Alex Schomburg's "The Conquest of Yellow Fever," Rudy Palais's "Walter Reed: The Man who Conquered Yellow Fever," and Nathan Schachner's "Healer of Men—A True Story of a Great Scientist."

Towards the end of the 1940s, Entertaining Comics (EC) appealed to the sentiments of the post-war era through themes of horror and violence, which in turn fermented anti-comics sentiments. Prominent critics of the genre then included a German-American psychiatrist, Fredric Wertham, who authored the *Seduction of the Innocent*, which blatantly censures comic reading based on his impressionistic clinical observations on human psychology. Wertham deduced that "chronic stimulation, temptation and seduction by comic books ... are contributing factors to many children's maladjustments" (490) and juvenile delinquency, which were rampant in the post-war America. Wertham's text incited several public demonstrations against comics, which eventually led to the inception of Comic Code Authority (CCA) by the Comics Magazine Association of America (CMAA) in 1954 (Gardner 102). The CCA applied stringent censorship on comic content, thereby forcing publishers and artists to restrain from portraying themes of bloodshed and violence (103). Thus, the silver age (1956–1969) witnessed a proliferation of a distinct genre of comics that dealt with non-controversial and facile themes (Roeder 7).

However, a countercultural movement originated in San Francisco during the mid-1960s, which was known as underground comics, or commix. According to Jared Gardner, artists like Robert Crumb, Jay Lynch, Skip Williamson, Gilbert Shelton, Denis Kitchen, and Art Spiegelman were the leading figures in the movement (115). Mostly aimed at challenging the norms of CCA, they explored taboo themes such as gender, sexuality, race, and drug addiction among other things, which were starkly distinct from the themes explored in traditional comic books (Gardner 125). Andrew J. Kunka established the spirit of counterculture in underground commix by stating that they were "defined by their resistance to censorship and the cultural norms of the time" and by "flaunt[ing] taboos often for the sake of exposing otherwise forbidden topics" (33). With their amateur publishing experience, underground comic artists revolutionised the form and content of the medium primarily through auto/biographies. As Williams contends, these works "represented a gradual shift in focus away from the exploits of heroic archetypes and towards the 'self' as the subject, rejecting orderly script structures in favour of entertaining chronicles of misadventures, confessions and chaotic vignettes from the hip community" (69). Celebrated commix magazines like *ZAP Comix, Help!, Bijou Funnies*, and *Mad* thus engaged in explicit, unorthodox portrayals of the human body. In so doing, underground comic artists established an unprecedented milieu for unabashed conversations about the body, illness, and sexuality through comics.

Accordingly, underground commix could be read as a primary movement towards the growth of personal narratives on healthcare quandaries. Justin Green's *Binky Brown Meets the Holy Virgin Mary* (hereafter *Binky Brown*) is often read as a meditation on sexuality and as the first extended confessional autobiographical comics (Venkatesan and Saji, "Royal Road" 170). Published in the underground in 1972, *Binky Brown* is an autobiographical graphic memoir concerned with Binky Brown's (Green's comic alter ego) Catholic guilt, sexual awakening, and struggles with obsessive compulsive disorder (OCD).

Green thoroughly exploits the immense potential of the medium in drawing the contours of his external and internal world that plagued him. Kunka argues that by utilising a symbolic/allegorical style as a method of autobiographical expression, Green literalises his fears and obsessions in the memoir (36). Quickly following suit, several comic artists of the time (especially those who belonged to the underground commix movement) produced their own short autobiographical accounts, thus expanding the new genre of comics. As Hillary Chute argues, *Binky Brown* is a "hugely influential text [which transformed] comics as a medium of self-expression" (14) and consequently led to the growth of personal narratives in the medium of comics.

## Narratives of Illness and the Birth of Graphic Medicine

As the demand for scientific objectivity and precision dominated medical discourse and as the ideological chasm between expert medical knowledge and individuals' unvoiced experiential knowledge widened, an attempt to formulate a humanist approach emerged around the 1970s to democratise medical practice and productively improve doctor-patient interactions (Charon, "Narrative Medicine" 1898). Rita Charon, who inaugurated this approach, christened it 'narrative medicine,' defining it as a "clinical cousin of literature-and-medicine and a literary cousin of relationship-centred care" (*Narrative Medicine* vii). As a holistic approach towards the expression of illness experiences and as a reaction against the oppressive absolutism of medical knowledge, according to Charon, narrative medicine provides "health care professionals with practical wisdom in comprehending what patients endure in illness and what they themselves undergo in the care of the sick" (*Narrative Medicine* vii). With the purpose of sharing and validating affective truths about illness and suffering, narrative medicine emphasises the phenomenological and intimate aspects of illness-related experiences. In effect, narrative medicine, while emphasising the need to integrate tacit knowledge into medical diagnosis and treatment, also underscores the need to acknowledge the sufferer's voice.

In "What to Do with Stories: The Sciences of Narrative Medicine," Charon clearly states that narrative medicine "refer[s] to clinical practice fortified by narrative competence—the capacity to recognize, absorb, metabolize, interpret, and be moved by stories of illness" (1265). Predictably, the proponents of narrative medicine, particularly Charon and Sayantani DasGupta, problematised the prescriptive nature of medical knowledge, in that they not only exposed the limitations and the vested authority of expert knowledge but also expanded a range of medical objectives and practices in paving a new way of understanding patients' subjectivity and relationships. DasGupta attests to exhorting the medical hierarchy to cultivate the culture of listening with 'narrative humility' where health professionals understand that

> stories are relationships [they] can approach and engage with while simultaneously remaining open to their ambiguity and contradiction and while engaging in constant self- evaluation and self-critique about issues such as [their] own role in the story as listeners, [their] expectations of the story, [their] responsibilities to the story, and [their] ownership of the story.
>
> (par. 13)

As an offshoot of this diverse and novel approach to the arts, literature, and medicine, graphic medicine ushered in new modes to address the tribulations and trauma of illness and thus articulated, according to Susan Merrill Squier, "aspects of social experience that escape[d] both the normal realms of medicine and the comforts of canonical literature" ("Literature" 130). Williams in the seminal indenture *Graphic Medicine Manifesto* observes this correlation of graphic medicine to the aims of narrative medicine thus: "graphic medicine combines the principles of narrative medicine with an exploration of the visual systems of comic art, interrogating the representation of physical and emotional signs and symptoms within the medium" (Czerwiec et al. 1). Put differently, graphic medicine, by utilising creative license and the diverse elements of the medium of comics, allows readers to explore multiple meanings of illness and disease, and, in so doing, it improvises the major premises of narrative medicine as it "opens up a space for thinking, being, and doing" (Diedrich 2).

## Preface to Graphic Medicine

The term 'graphic medicine' was coined by the British physician and comic artist, Dr Ian Williams in 2007, introducing an interdisciplinary field that explores the "personal side of medicine, instead of the physiology and the mechanics" (Janbazian) of a specific disease. The *Graphic Medicine Manifesto,* which was published in 2015, integrates scholarly essays by the founders of graphic medicine (viz. MK Czerwiec, Williams, Squier, Michael J. Green, Kimberly R. Myers, and Scott T. Smith); a few comic narratives on illness; and several short personal endorsements of the significance of graphic medicine by several artists, scholars, and patients. Such a framework further illustrates what the *Manifesto* proposes: "graphic medicine resists the notion of the universal patient and vividly represents multiple subjects with valid and, at times, conflicting points of view and experiences" (Czerwiec et al. 2). Essentially, the inherent propensity of graphic medicine to authentically document a myriad of perspectives evinces a nuanced understanding of illness and healthcare quandaries as experienced by the patients, doctors, and caregivers. Integrating images and texts, graphic pathography—or illness narratives in the form of comics—has emerged as a "distinctive sub-genre of graphic stories" (Green and Myers 574), intending to reduce the chasm between doctors and patients. Despite the fact that graphic pathographies and textual illness narratives discuss similar thematic concerns, the "powerful visual messages [of graphic pathographies] convey an immediate visceral understanding in ways that conventional texts cannot" (574). These artists, in their illness narratives, often create new iconography for a particular illness or refashion the existing symbols in accordance with their subjective experience. Either way, what they do enhances the visual expressivity of an illness and dismantles negative stereotypes that surround a particular disease. Also, graphic pathographers' avant-garde style of depicting subjective illness experience democratises the verbo-visual discourse of medicine that was earlier monopolised by doctors and medical illustrators. Additionally, the potential of graphic medical narratives to depict the complex subjective experience by deploying the affordances of comics such as spatio-temporality, economy of expression, and gestures makes it a safe space for discussing sensitive issues.

Such multifarious features that are unique to the medium of comics provide a leeway to combine, what Czerweic et al. call, "subjective feelings and perceptions with the objective visual representation" (19). First, the aesthetic as well as the visual nuances make comics a productive juncture that joins the author and the reader onto the same plane as the reader actively engages in generating meaning across the panels through what McCloud refers to as "closure" (65). Temporal flexibility and the lack of spatial strictures aid the artists in depicting the permanence as well as the transcendence of time, which is pivotal in illness narratives to depict, what Henri Bergson calls, psychic time and objective time (qtd. in El Refaie, *Autobiographical* 96). In a different way, assenting the depictions of a near-to-life appeal, gestures make comics more dynamic through the careful relaying of human emotions (Venkatesan and Saji, "Rhetorics" 226). Replicating the interplay of emotions through images and reinforcing their impact through the affordance of gestures, comics guide pathographers in mirroring moments that are too expressive for verbal narration. While making visible the intricate intrapsychic experiences of illnesses, the genre of comics allows artists a unique opportunity to reincarnate themselves into the intradiegetic realms of the narrative through embodiment. On the other hand, validating as it were, the narrative's truthfulness leaves the subjective marks of the author as an asseveration of the autobiographical pact. Put differently, the exhaustiveness of all these attributes makes comics highly expressive yet succinct, and thus an ideal medium to represent illness experiences.

Second, illness experiences thus delineated through the medium of comics are therefore potent verbo-visual transcriptions of intense intra-subjective and phenomenological truths that are often disaccredited by medical knowledge and its attendant epistemology. As Green asserts, "comics can give voice to the unsettling worries and concerns that may be difficult to articulate through words alone" ("Comics and Medicine" 774). Blending verbal and visual semiotic codes, comics allow the author to express an idiosyncratic and intricately embodied experience in a universal way, thereby inviting the readers to the author's visceral and immediate experiences. Since trauma occasioned by illness is untranslatable, comics embody such tacit impressions, providing better ways of negotiating illness experiences. Comics, as Squier attests, "direct our attention to the meaning conveyed by the body and its movements, gestures, and postures" (Czerwiec et al. 49). Coupled with the McCloudian notion of closure, the formal attributes make comics the ideal medium for narrating the tacit experiences of illness and disabilities. Consequently, comics facilitate artists in recreating their illness experiences in a visceral and immediate manner to reclaim their experiences. In essence, the structural singularity and formal attributes of the medium not only extend ingress into the subjective realities of other sufferers but also enable both cognitive and sensual perceptions of the otherwise ineffable intricacies of human lives.

## Graphic Pathographies

Graphic pathographies (illness narratives in comic form) often portray experiences pertaining to physical illness, mental illness, and disability. Justin Green's *Binky Brown,* which poignantly discloses the artist's private shame regarding his OCD, is often referred to as the first graphic pathography. Art Spiegelman in the Introduction to *Binky Brown* referred to it as a "forty-four page … epic" in which Green depicts his psychic angst by incorporating numerous visual metaphors and experimenting with the formal features of comics such as panels, borders, layouts, and lettering. Subsequently, Al Davison's 1991 publication *The Spiral Cage: Diary of An Astral Gypsy* (hereafter *The Spiral Cage*) documents Davison's experience of living with spina bifida. Deploying the technique of chiaroscuro, Davison captures the indignation that he suffered as an orthopedically abnormal child and his encounter with Buddhist ideals that enabled him to confront his disability with resilience. Written ahead of their time, both *Binky Brown* and *The Spiral Cage* were unrecognised by the mainstream literature until the post-millennial era, when literature began celebrating the synergy between comics and healthcare (Beaty and Woo 23).

Heralding the distinctive features of comics to the mainstream audience, Harvey Pekar and Joyce Brabner's autopathography *Our Cancer Year*, published in 1994, poignantly narrates Pekar's struggles with lymphoma and Brabner's perspectives on caring for him. In order to present a holistic experience of illness and caregiving, Pekar and Brabner integrated sub-plots into their memoir that focussed on the political upheavals of the Gulf War around which their personal lives were revolving. Thereafter, numerous graphic pathographies popularised the discourse of graphic medicine and reinforced the potency of this form. These include such works as Judd Winick's *Pedro and Me: Friendship, Loss, and What I Learned*, in which Winick meditates on his caregiving experience and the stigma that his friend Pedro encountered as a person living with AIDS; Samuel C. Williams' *At War with Yourself*, in which Williams narrates his friend Matt's struggle with PTSD; and Alison Bechdel's *Fun Home: A Family Tragicomic* which records Bechdel's negotiation with her OCD and lesbian identity, among other things.

Autopathographies such as David Small's *Stitches: A Memoir* and Brick's *Depresso: How I Learned to Stop Worrying and Embrace Being Bonkers!* provide a subjective account of throat cancer and depression, respectively, in shades of black and white. Both these artists, by pictorially narrating their illness experiences, critique the "epistemological authority of the medical profession" (Squier and Marks 150) through unique visual iconography. In addition to dealing with psychosomatic illness, graphic pathographies also deal with experiences with injury and disability. Some of the notable graphic disability narratives are Kaisa Leka's *I am Not These Feet*, in which Leka recounts her trauma after the amputation of her feet, and Chris Ware's *The Acme Novelty Library 18,* in which Ware narrates the life of a young girl after her below-the-knee amputation. In short, graphic pathographies analyse "a range of issues broadly termed 'medical'" (Czerwiec et al. cover), which grants voice to hitherto marginalised perspectives on illness.

## Are Graphic Pathographies Education Comics?

The difference between graphic medical narratives and medical educational comics is significant in delineating the scope of graphic medicine in the domains of art, literature, and medicine. Medical educational comics are a sub-cluster of graphic medicine that aims at providing patients and caregivers with factual details about a specific disease (Farinella). Alternatively, graphic medical narratives emphasise vocalising experiences with subjective illnesses. An in-group distinction between these two narrative forms of graphic medicine facilitates a lucid understanding of pathographies on mental illness that will be discussed in this dissertation. Although educational comics play a pivotal role in creating awareness of mental illness and providing reassurance to the sufferers, in the present study, educational comics are not examined; rather, graphic pathographies on mental illness are explored for its eminent literariness. Akin to numerous mainstream auto/biographical texts, graphic medical narratives rely on sharing experiences with their readers. In reconstructing the artists' lived experiences, these graphic pathographers experiment with avant-garde art styles and thereby create a uniquely rich verbo-visual vocabulary to discuss the ineffable and complex experience of illness.

Educational comics often follow simplistic and illustrative art styles as they are crafted with pedagogical intent aimed at a particular target group. Used by public health professionals, NGOs, and government agencies, these comics discuss health-related issues in third person narration with clinical precision. Joshua Cadwell defines educational comics as a "subset of comics whose purpose is not to tell a story or to entertain but to transfer information and communicate concepts" (qtd. in McNicol 20). Utilised as a pedagogic tool in the healthcare system, these narratives cater to a definitive target audience with limited cognitive and linguistic skills. For example, Kirsti Evans and John Swogger's *Something Different About Dad: How to Live with Your Asperger's Parent* educates children between 7 and 15 years old about Asperger syndrome and suggests various adapting techniques to accommodate the idiosyncrasies of an Asperger parent. No different is Ed Hillyer's *Love S.T.I.ngs: A Beginner's Guide to Sexually Transmitted Infections,* which aims to create sexual health awareness and safe sex practices among teenagers. As these texts signal to their readers the possible predicaments of a particular disease and assist them in the process of managing sicknesses, educational comics function as a practical guide for sufferers and for caregivers. Graphic pathographies such as David B's *Epileptic*, on the other hand, explore complex themes of subjective illness experiences in creative ways, modulating angle, colour, frame, and background. Unlike educational comics, the narrative structure of these pathographies varies from writer to writer. Devoid of a definitive beginning, middle, and end, comic authors narrate their experience in order to gain purgation and to create a community for themselves through empathetic readers. The dynamics of word and image in these comics are far more complex than in most educational comics. Here, the image and text can either complement or supplement each other, and still at other times, act independently of each other.

## Graphic Medicine as a Critique of Biomedicine

As Squier and Marks observe in the introduction to *Configurations*, graphic medicine provides new perspectives, highlights "the disruptive urgency of graphic memoirs," questions the "epistemological authority of medical profession," exposes the healthcare professional's 'personal vulnerability,' and presents medical technologies in a different perspective as well (150). In so doing, graphic medicine "provides an easy alternative to confronting the actual emotional and physical vulnerability and pain" (150). Graphic medicine gains its import when individuals' voices find a community and gain acceptance as a valid differential knowledge. Comics evolved out of the experiences of medical practitioners who have divulged their 'emotional vulnerability' as well as their struggles with institutional medicine provide ingress to those illness experiences that have been taboo (Venkatesan and Peter 198).

When mainstream literature and medical humanities glorified the vocation of a physician as quasi divine, not much speculation was done in weighing out the degree of truth in it (Venkatesan and Peter 189). However, physicians started to express their private selves, especially through the medium of comics, that many times physicians are in dire need of care, and there are doctors who are ostracised by their own community. In a way, as Brady et al. remark, graphic medicine "allows clinicians to realize that they bring into each encounter their whole selves: their physical beings, their emotions, their strengths and their weaknesses" (qtd. in Fong 275).

Breaking physicians' silence among the clamour of mainstream literature's depictions of their fraternity, physicians in graphic medicine comics have exposed themselves as vulnerable beings, who are not pretending to be courageous, composed, and considerate. Graphic medicine thus, according to Nick Sousanis, offers "a kaleidoscopic view [that] serves to shift our vision from one dimension to a more multi-dimensional view" that connects varying voices together in "a rhizomatic structure" (39). Re-structuring the glorified capabilities of physicians, pathographies like *The Bad Doctor, Missed It, Betty. P, Stitches*, and *Epileptic* project doctors from a different vantage point, which destabilises the popular expectations of doctors by projecting their humanity and vulnerability. In a conversation with Deborah Bowman, Ian Williams explains how he "found the 'voice'" in comics to talk about being stigmatised since he was a physician who was an OCD patient as well.

Graphic medicine as a countercultural discourse intercepts this monopoly of medical knowledge by validating and prioritising the patients' lived experiences. In so doing, the genre not only endorses multiple ways of dealing with illness but also facilitates empathy and creates awareness of a particular disease. For instance, departing from the existing binaries of triumphalism and sentimentalising, in her graphic memoir *Cancer Made Me a Shallower Person,* Miriam Engelberg enunciates a philosophy of 'shallowness' and creates a new way of dealing with breast cancer. Likewise, in her graphic memoir *Lighter Than My Shadow*, Katie Green re-orients the popular under-standing of an eating disorder due to body image, gender, sexuality, and trauma.

The strength of graphic medicine, according to Sousanis, lies in the "simultaneous engagement of multiple vantage points from which to engender new ways of seeing" (32). In valuing the patients', caregivers', and vulnerable doctors' voices, graphic medicine exists as a non-hegemonic form of knowledge by accommodating multiplicity, plurality, and polysemy. Hence, a productive tension exists between what Moreno-Leguizamon et al. call "epistemological world-views of social sciences and humanities" and the "personal, relational, ethical, and moral value competencies" in graphic medicine (18, 22). Unlike the scientific epistemology which tend to suppress sufferers' voices, graphic medicine becomes more productive, in that it refuses to silence any voices. Doctors, patients, and caregivers exist on the same panel for the readers to ponder over and react to the ideologies that conceal and silence the vulnerable. For instance, Stan Mack's graphic memoir *Janet and Me: An Illustrated Story of Love and Loss* is a suitable example to demonstrate how graphic medicine puts together individual narratives. The memoir diegetically accommodates the multiple voices of Janet's doctors, friends, nurses, neighbours, nurses, and family members along with Mack's own account of Janet. In representing time spatially, comics documents the experience 'in synchronic time' as well as it provides what Squier refers to as "narrative access to diachronic time" (Czerwiec et al. 46). The democratic medium of comics with its multiple formal possibilities connects and prompts the reflection of intricate relationships among doctors, patients, and caregivers.

## From Book Stalls to Classrooms

As the irrefutable power of comics was established in science educational programs in steering the public towards healthy lifestyle practices, narratives of illness experience are being used in medical schools to help future doctors develop healthy relationships with patients and develop clinical skills. Since 2009, at the Penn State Milton S. Hershey Medical Center, Michael Green has been offering an elective course on "Graphic Storytelling and Medical Narratives" based on three major objectives: to

> 1) expose students to a set of medically relevant graphic narratives that provoke critical reflection about the experience of illness and the ways patients and their families interface with the medical system; 2) equip students with critical thinking skills for reading and understanding comics that are relevant to medical practice; and 3) nurture students' creativity by helping them develop their own stories into original graphic narratives.
>
> ("Teaching with" 472)

As part of the course, the fourth-year medical students are introduced to different graphic pathographies like Ken Dahl's *Monsters*, Joyce Farmer's *Special Exits*, and Thom Ferrier's *Disrepute*, among others. Later, they are asked to deliberate and reflect on the issues that are discussed in these graphic pathographies. At the end of the course, medical students are required to create their own comics, and then these comic projects are displayed on the walls of the medical school and are also made available on the college website (476). Some of the popular works created include Ashley L. Pistorio's *Vita Perseverat* or *Life Goes On* and Taylor Olmsted's *The Taming of Tina*.

Czerwiec and Green observe that reading graphic medical narratives has significantly helped healthcare professionals to reflect and comprehend the healthcare issues that might not have been otherwise visible ("Mayo Clinic"). Interpreting graphic pathographies has encouraged medical students and practising doctors to be empathetic listeners and better clinicians. In their seminal essay, "Graphic Medicine: Use of Comics in Medical Education," Green and Myers assert that physicians can use graphic pathographies to describe and disentangle the process of diagnosis and prognosis of a particular disease to patients and caregivers, and most importantly, they also provide succour by "elicit[ing] the patient's treatment preferences" (576). While doctoring skills demand physicians to decode the symptoms of patients from sometimes incoherent narratives, medical history, and physical examination, reading the inherently fragmented narrative of comics will facilitate healthcare providers to enhance their critical thinking and diagnostic reasoning (Czerwiec et al. 73).

Creation of comics, according to Green, grants medical students "the freedom to reflect honestly (and safely) about the forces that shape their emerging professional identities" (Green, "Comics and Medicine" 4). Drawing comics not only offers students a chance for creative expression in a highly taxing medical curriculum but also provides them a sense of agency in drafting their narrative. Meditating on their comic project allows students to explore numerous possibilities of communicating a specific issue. In so doing, they unconsciously develop better communicative strategies that would bridge the communicational chasm between doctors and patients during a clinical encounter. Additionally, comic creation provides students a "satisfaction in their accomplishments" (Czerwiec et al. 77). Mastery over a new medium in a short span bestows self-confidence in students and reduces the angst of isolation and depression that medical students encounter in their formative years.

Reading, discussing, and creating graphic pathographies offer interns a space to articulate their suffering and stress-related crises in clinical settings. In narratives like Ryan Montoya's *Sign Out* and Michael Natter's *Code Blue*, the authors discuss the helplessness, conflicts, and fears that medical students harbour within them. In her essay, "Graphic Medicine in the University," Squier highlights a response from Josh, an English graduate who remarks that "[t]he medical education that graphic medicine provides can be useful for healing and for prevention of psychological injuries by fostering resilience" (22) in medical students. Graphic pathographies expedite medical practitioners' surmounting what Czerwiec and Green call "narrative constipation" or the "stuffing down" ("Mayo Clinic") of emotionally fraught stories within a healthcare provider. According to Czerwiec and Green, doctors' and medical students' suppressing and neglecting themselves will eventually threaten their own physical and mental well-being.

Untranslatable emotions and feelings of guilt that most physicians suppress and hide find a leeway for expression in reading and creating comics (Venkatesan and Peter 198). For instance, in his comic article titled "Missed It" published in the *Annals of Internal Medicine* in 2013, Green apolitically discusses his diagnostic error and guilt over relying on another doctor's assessment rather than trusting his own instincts which eventually leads to the death of his patient when he was an intern. The subversive nature and the innate levity of the medium of comics facilitated Green's initiating a placid discussion of an otherwise controversial theme. Reiterating similar concerns, Darren B. Taichman, executive deputy editor of the *Annals of Internal Medicine,* states that the "graphic novel might provide a safe place where people feel comfortable expressing...uncomfortable issues" (qtd. in Glazer 16). In the graphic narratives of healthcare providers such as Ian Williams' *The Bad Doctor: The Troubled Life and Times of Dr Iwan James*, Green's *Betty. P*, Czerwiec's *Taking Turns: Stories From HIV/AIDS Care Unit 371*, and Grace E. Farris's *Anatomy of a Donut Hole,* the authors recount the doctors' and interns' helplessness during medical training and practice.

## Trends in Graphic Medicine

Graphic pathographies are mostly published by individual artists who focus on delineating the phenomenological dimensions of illness. These comic narratives about experiences of illness are either drawn by the sufferers themselves or co-authored by illustrators who help the sufferers to visualise the contours of inexplicable pain. Apart from print publishers like Astral Gypsy, Fantagraphics, SelfMadeHero, and Abrams ComicArts, which produce critically acclaimed graphic novels and graphic memoirs on illness experiences, a range of independent artists utilise the internet to create and share their unique experiences of illness. Many of the popular graphic pathographies on cancer and depression, such as Brian Fies' *Mom's Cancer* and Allie Brosh's *Hyperbole and a Half*, were originally published as webcomics. Upon overwhelming positive reception to these works, the serialised comics were subsequently published in print. Several other pathographers continue to use webcomics' potential to effectively translate their physical and mental health issues. In his webcomic *These Memories Won't Last,* for instance, Stu Campbell explores the possibilities of animation and sound in telling the story of his grandfather's decline into dementia. The words and images on the screen appear and soon disappear, unable to be scrolled back up to review, in a way simulating the experience of losing memory. The comments section available in webcomics further engages readers in forming a community of sufferers who identify with the authors' illnesses. Over 5,000 comments, which Brosh received on her blog "Hyperbole and a Half," bear witness to a global recognition and acceptance of the medium of comics as suitable for expressing personal perspectives on illness. With the onset of the COVID-19 pandemic, several artists (such as Rachael House, Malcolm Mayes, and Mike Natter, among others) have explored the possibilities of the digital medium to examine issues such as bioethics, healthcare services, coping, and healthcare disparities, among others.

Fies' *Mom's Cancer*, a graphic memoir about caring for his mother who was suffering from lung cancer, became a seminal inspiration for the founders of graphic medicine to constitute the graphic medicine collective ("Mayo Clinic"). Later, *Mom's Cancer* was translated into German, French, Italian, and Japanese due to its impact on the community of patients, caregivers, and healthcare professionals like Czerwiec. Although several such graphic pathographies are illustrated and published professionally, graphic medicine also encourages amateur artists to draw their unique experiences of illness, which could engage readers in a more intimate fashion. Drawing inspiration from the website graphicmedicine.org which grants access to reviews, scholarly essays, and primary sources on graphic medicine, groups of like-minded artists/scholars/healthcare professionals have initiated similar website/association in Spain and Japan. Led by physician and comics artist Monica Lalanda, *Medicina Grafica* is a graphic medicine website for Spanish readers. Similarly, the Japan Graphic Medicine Association (JGMA) has become a global forum for exchanging ideas related to graphic medicine. Graphic medicine also rose to popularity in Taiwan with the publication of *Crazy Hospital* in 2013, which details sarcastic caricatures of hospital culture in Taiwan. Created by a psychiatrist, Dr Tse-yao Lin, and illustrated by graphic artist, Liang Yuan, *Crazy Hospital* inspired Taiwanese medical practitioners to express themselves through comics. Detailing their experiences in medical school and their interactions with patients, Taiwanese doctors promote and publicise their works in social media platforms like Facebook. In India, though graphic medicine is in its nascence, an online graphic medicine group called 'Comicos' at the University College of Medical Sciences, Delhi, and the Graphic Medicine Lab under the aegis of Sathyaraj Venkatesan at the National Institute of Technology, Trichy, are noteworthy.

Due to the increasing popularity of graphic narratives on illness, several artists have been choosing to adapt these memoirs into other media. Sarah Leavitt's graphic memoir about her mother's Alzheimer's disease, *Tangles: A Story About Alzheimer's, My Mother and Me*, is being adapted to a feature length animation by Giant Ant Media. The trailer features background narration, music, and visual effects to Leavitt's original drawings. Similarly, Czerwiec's recent memoir, *Taking Turns: Stories from HIV/AIDS Care Unit 371*, was adapted as a staged reading by Duke Theatre Studies Professor Dr Jules Odendahl-James and the undergraduates in her Spring 2017 class, "Medical Stories on Stage."

## Conclusion

Comics' engagement with healthcare dates back to the national dailies of the 1860s, which featured numerous public health-related caricatures. Prompted by the dissatisfaction towards the government and entrepreneurs' exploitative approaches towards marginal communities, these cartoons primarily vocalised the public's frustration about inadequate national healthcare facilities. Later, in the 1920s, comics engaged with themes of fantasy and idealism, which percolated from superheroes to scientists and doctors. In the post-war era, the theme of medical comics shifted from hagiographies to mundane experiences of healthcare professionals within clinical settings. Subsequently, in the 1960s, with the onset of an underground comics movement, a subversive wave took over personal disclosures about health and illness. Seminal works such as Green's *Binky Brown,* Kominsky-Crumb's "Goldie: A Neurotic Woman," and Spiegelman's *Maus* refashioned the stylistic and thematic proclivities of comics towards subjective spaces. Drawing inspiration from the commix artists, countless cartoonists started discussing their personal healthcare predicaments through comics.

Taking cues from these historic roots, graphic medicine exposes the vulnerable aspects of healthcare and illness for a productive change in clinical encounters. Situated at the crossroads of comics and medicine, graphic medicine aims to promote patients', caregivers', and doctors' affective knowledge and subjective truths. Departing from the monolithic biomedical approach towards patient identity and healthcare prescriptions, these graphic pathographies make visible both patients' and doctors' otherwise unvoiced emotions. In doing so, an alternative body of medical knowledge emerges in graphic medicine, one which promotes a holistic attitude towards healing and formulates a community of sufferers who identify with each other's personal experiences.

## Reference List

Beaty, Bart, and Benjamin Woo. *The Greatest Comic Book of All Time: Symbolic Capital and the Field of American Comic Books*. Palgrave, 2016.

Bowman, Deborah. "Patients and Doctors Now Draw on Their Experience to Provide a 'Comic-Strip' View of Illness." The Conversation, 1 July 2014, https://theconversation.com/patients-and-doctors-now-draw-on-their-experience-to-provide-a-comic-strip-view-of-illness-25515.

Charon, Rita. "Narrative Medicine: A Model for Empathy, Reflection, Profession, and Trust." *JAMA*, vol. 286, no. 15, 2001, pp. 1897–1902.

———. *Narrative Medicine: Honoring the Stories of Illness*. Oxford UP, 2006.

———. "What to Do with Stories: The Sciences of Narrative Medicine." *Canadian Family Physician*, vol. 53, no. 8, 2007, pp. 1265–1267.

Chute, Hillary. *Graphic Women: Life Narrative and Contemporary Comics*. Columbia UP, 2010.

Czerwiec, M. K., et al. *Graphic Medicine Manifesto*. The Pennsylvania State UP, 2015.

DasGupta, Sayantani. "Narrative Medicine, Narrative Humility: Listening to the Streams of Stories." *Creative Nonfiction: True Stories, Well Told*, no. 52, 2014. https://www.creativenonfiction.org/online-reading/narrative-medicine-narrative-humility.

Diedrich, Lisa. *Treatment: Language, Politics, and the Culture of Illness*. U of Minnesota P, 2007.

El Refaie, Elisabeth. *Autobiographical Comics: Life Writing in Pictures*. UP of Mississippi, 2012.

Farinella, Matteo. "Science Comics' Super Powers." *American Scientist*, vol. 106, no. 4, 2018. doi: 10.1511/2018.106.4.218

Fong, Harmon. "Medthics Graphic Novel." *Journal of Medical Humanities*, vol. 33, no. 4, 2012, pp. 273–285.

Gardner, Jared. *Projections: Comics and the History of the Twenty-first-century Storytelling*. Stanford UP, 2012.

Glazer, Sarah. "Graphic Medicine: Comics Turn a Critical Eye on Health Care." *Hastings Center Report*, vol. 45, no. 3, 2015, pp. 15–19.

Green, Justin. *Binky Brown Meets the Holy Virgin Mary*. McSweeney's, 2009.

Green, Michael J. "Comics and Medicine: Peering into the Process of Professional Identity Formation." *Academic Medicine*, vol. 90, no. 6, 2015, pp. 774–779.

———. "Teaching with Comics: A Course for Fourth-Year Medical Students." *Journal of Medical Humanities*, vol. 34, no. 4, 2013, pp. 471–476.

Green, Michael J., and Kimberly R. Myers. "Graphic Medicine: Use of Comics in Medical Education and Patient Care." *BMJ*, vol. 340, 2010, pp. 574–577.

Hansen, Bert. "Medical History for the Masses: How American Comic Books Celebrated Heroes of Medicine in the 1940s." *Bulletin of the History of Medicine*, no. 78, 2004, pp. 148–191.

———. "The Image and Advocacy of Public Health in American Caricature and Cartoons from 1860 to 1900." *American Journal of Public Health*, vol. 87, no. 11, 1997, pp. 1798–1807.

Janbazian, Rupen. "Lyricism, Magic, and Graphic Medicine: An Interview with Dana Walrath." The Armenian Weekly, 20 November 2015, https://armenianweekly.com/2015/11/20/between-palu-and-ny/.

Kunka, Andrew. *Autobiographical Comics*. Bloomsbury Academic, 2018.

Kunzle, David. *Father of the Comic Strip: Rodolph Töpffer*. UP of Mississippi, 2007.

Mainardi, Patricia. "The Invention of Comics." *Nineteenth-Century Art Worldwide*, vol. 6, no. 1, 2007, pp. 1–18.

"Mayo Clinic Transform 2013 Symposium, "INSIGHTS" with MK Czerwiec and Michael Green, M.D." YouTube, uploaded by Mayo Clinic, 16 October 2013, https://www.youtube.com/watch?v=zTRvoQGBs0Y.

McCloud, Scott. *Understanding Comics: The Invisible Art*. Harper Perennial, 1994.

McNicol, Sarah. "The Potential of Educational Comics as a Health Information Medium." *Health Information and Libraries Journal*, no. 34, 2016, pp. 20–31. https://onlinelibrary.wiley.com/doi/epdf/10.1111/hir.12145.

Moreno-Leguizamon, Carlos J. et al. "Incorporation of Social Sciences and Humanities in the Training of Health Professionals and Practitioners in Other Ways of Knowing." *RHiME*, vol. 2, 2015, pp. 18–23.

Roeder, Joshua R. Silver Age Comic Books: Uncovering their Importance in the Midst of Political, Social, and Cultural Movements of the 1960s and 1970s. 2013. Wichita State U, MA Dissertation.

Sousanis, Nick. *Unflattening*. Harvard University Press, 2015.

Squier, Susan M. "Graphic Medicine in the University." *Hastings Centre Report*, no. 3, 2015, pp. 19–22.

———. "Literature and Medicine, Future Tense: Making it Graphic." *Literature and Medicine*, vol. 27, no. 1, 2009, pp. 124–152.

Squier, Susan M., and J. Ryan Marks. "Introduction." *Configurations*, vol. 22, no. 2, 2014, pp. 149–152.

Venkatesan, Sathyaraj, and Anu Mary Peter. "No Time to Rest, Vent or Mourn: Medical Intern Narratives and Graphic Medicine." *Inks: The Journal of the Comics Studies Society*, vol. 1, no. 2, 2017, pp. 186–204.

Venkatesan, Sathyaraj, and Sweetha Saji. "Rhetorics of the Visual: Graphic Medicine, Comics and its Affordances." *Rupkatha Journal on Interdisciplinary Studies in Humanities*, vol. 8, no. 3, 2016, pp. 221–231.

———. "Royal Road to Wisdom: Tarot Cards and Justin Green's Binky Brown Meets the Holy Virgin Mary." *The Explicator*, vol. 74, no. 3, 2016, pp. 170–172.

Wertham, Fredric. "Such Trivia as Comic Books." *The Children's Culture Reader*, edited by Henry Jenkins, New York UP, 1999, pp. 486–493.

Williams, Ian. "Graphic Medicine: The Portrayal of Illness in Underground and Autobiographical Comics." *Medicine, Health and the Arts: Approaches to the Medical Humanities*, edited by Victoria Bates et al., Routledge, 2014, pp. 64–84.

# 2 Function of Metaphors in Illness Narratives

## Introduction

With changing literary and socio-cultural conventions, theories on metaphor have undergone revision in their conceptualisation and use since Aristotle's *Poetics*. Although Aristotle premised his theoretical framework of metaphor on analogy, most contemporary research on metaphor is grounded on its role as a linguistic device and of poetic imagination until the radical exploratory studies made by George Lakoff and Mark Johnson, who redefined metaphor as a characteristic of thought and action. However, a systematic reflection on metaphor as a phenomenon of lived experience and conditions for its expression is lacking in different metaphor theories. Therefore, this chapter will provide an overview of the major theoretical postulates on metaphor, with an emphasis on Lakoff and Johnson's conceptual metaphor theory (CMT) since the implications of the theory correspond to the objectives of the study. Further, the wider implications of using metaphors, especially visual metaphors in autobiographical graphic pathographies, will be analysed in the context of illness.

Originating from the theories of Greek philosophers like Plato, Aristotle, and Cicero, metaphors were understood as a matter of language, not thought. This classical theory of metaphor proposed that metaphorical expressions were mutually exclusive from the realm of everyday literal language. Based on similarities, two concepts were compared in rhetoric intended for aesthetic qualities such as "rhetorical force and stylistic vividness and pleasantness of a discourse" (Abrams 155). Juxtaposition of classical metaphor theory with Lakoff and Johnson's cognitive approach to metaphors of the twentieth century reflects a definitive paradigm shift from locating metaphors as a matter of words/language to a matter of thought/action. However, this

DOI: 10.4324/9781003214229-3

perspectival shift was shaped across the centuries of theorising metaphors in literary and philosophical domains.

## A Brief Outline of Metaphor Theories

### Comparison Theory

Aristotle's view of metaphor as an implicit comparison, based on analogy and its aesthetic function, forms the basis of the comparison theory of metaphors. According to this theory (also called similarity theory), a metaphor is understood by comparing its two constituent terms to find its common features. In other words, comparison theory views metaphor as an implicit simile. Unlike similes, which are comparisons made explicit by the use of the terms 'as' or 'like,' comparison theory asserts the truth value of a metaphor by listing all respects of their similarities. Max Black states that a "metaphor consists in the presentation of the underlying analogy or similarity" to its literal equivalent (283). In other words, Black calls this view of metaphors a "condensed or elliptical simile" (283). Although this view surmises the traditional persuasive and decorative function of metaphors, it overrides the distinction between comparison and categorisation. As Cacciari contends, the entities of a metaphor have in common "more than mere resemblances in that they belong to the same category sharing relevant features" (135–136). Here, rather than constructing similarities between two distinct entities, the author merely correlates two concepts that are already associated by possible experience. The shared features of a metaphor, according to comparison theory, are from a fixed set. Thus, in interpreting a metaphor, a common category must be found for the target and source, and the fixed feature sets must be activated from which identical features must be found. Comparison theory of metaphors also extends the argument towards the generation of novel associations between distinct entities with the correlation of existing similarities.

### Transference Theory

As one of the oldest theories of metaphor, transference theory is associated with Aristotle's characterisation of metaphor as a sign of absolute linguistic mastery. In locating the specific use of metaphor in poetry, Aristotle regarded metaphor as a decoration or ornament, not integral to the functioning of language. Aristotle defined metaphor as "transference of a term from one thing to another": the transference being either from "genus to species, species to genus, species to species, or by an analogy" (qtd. in Halliwell 55). In other words, when the reader/listener confronts something outside the ambit of usual language, resemblances that are transferred from one genus to species or vice versa, or between species of ideas, will deepen his/her experience and enrich his/her apprehension of the world. However, contemporary critics find Aristotle's definition problematic, in that he does not distinguish between metaphor and other tropes, such as metonymy, synecdoche, and irony, although metonymy (genus to species) and synecdoche (species to genus) are also contained in Aristotle's definition. As such, all forms of transference would count as figures of speech in general. Further distinction between the broad and narrow notions of metaphor has been suggested by semiotician Winfried Nöth according to whom the narrow notion of metaphor signifies metaphor as a particular figure of speech and the broad notion denoting all figures of speech as metaphors (128).

Aristotle's idea of metaphor fostered the misconception that the strangeness of metaphors is necessarily bound to rhetorics and not to the ordinary. However, later metaphor theories postulate that metaphors describe poetic aspects of everyday language instead of being considered as a predominant feature of poetic language. Aristotle also foregrounds the principle of analogy between two unrelated ideas in a metaphor. In his example for a metaphor—"the evening of life"—the analogy between evening and old age is determined by their similar proportions (qtd. in Kirby 534). Therefore, by these two principles of strangeness and analogy, the operation of metaphors converges the matters of similarity as well as dissimilarity.

The notion of transference implies metaphorically that the characteristics of one thing are transferred to another thing (Isenberg 610). In this comprehension of one matter in terms of another, critics problematise whether the transference is made possible due to a preexisting analogy or is claimed in their operation. Therefore, it leads to substitution where strangeness, analogy, and transference converge. Accordingly, in a metaphor, an ordinary expression is substituted with something non-ordinary (strange), implying the transference of meaning of one noun to another, which is possible only because of an existing analogy between both of them (Black 285). The reader thus engages in an act of deciphering the literal meaning of one noun using the literal meaning of the other as an indicator. This process of transference conglomerated with strangeness, analogy, and substitution incidentally remedies the gap in the literal vocabulary—thereby transforming metaphors as a 'species of *catachresis*' (Black 280) where common words gather new senses. Black argues, however, that when the catachrestic function of metaphor cannot be invoked, attempts at "substituting an indirect, metaphorical, expression are taken to be stylistic" (281).

### Interaction Theory

First advocated by the literary theorist I.A. Richards, interaction theory of metaphor holds that "thought is metaphoric, and proceeds by comparison, and the metaphors of language derive therefrom" (94). Here, metaphors operate by the interplay between the source and target of a metaphor as readers invent relationship between them to arrive at meaning. In introducing the terms *vehicle* for the metaphorical word and *tenor* for the subject to which the metaphorical word is applied, Richards proposed that a metaphor functions through the interaction between these, not by the similarities between them (100). Rather than being an embellishment to the tenor, a vehicle co-operates/interacts with it in generating a meaning distinct from either of the elements. Further, Richards posits that this interaction between tenor and vehicle can potentially create a metaphor dependent on an adequate context. Accordingly, metaphors are freely evoked instead of commonplace comparisons, in that the practicality of it will vary from one socio-cultural setting to another.

Refining and expanding I.A. Richards's interaction view of metaphors, Black proposed that the two elements of a metaphor—"subsidiary subject" (286) (Richards' 'vehicle') and "principal subject" (287) (Richards's 'tenor')—interacts along a "system of associated commonplaces" (287) whereby this complex set of associations serves to select and reorganise a "distinctive intellectual operation" (293) in the reader/listener in order to evoke new ways of perceiving the 'principal subject.' Black critiques the traditional view of metaphors as stylistic devices, arguing that the predominant function of metaphors is to "remedy a gap in the vocabulary" (280) and that a metaphor's effectiveness relies not on the authenticity of the comparison made but in the fact that their meanings may be freely evoked. Accordingly, Black documents three distinct views/theories of metaphors: (a) comparison view, (b) substitution view, and (c) interaction view (292). Endorsing the third view of metaphors, Black argues that here, the reader is forced naturally to connect the two distinct ideas—in other words, to use a system of associated commonplaces as the frame imposes extension of meaning upon context of the focal word (principal subject), thereby gathering a new meaning distinct from its literal use (287).

Since the interaction view proposes a distinctive mode of operation based on socio-cultural systems of implications, Black, who developed this idea, argues for the prerequisite of reader involvement in deciphering the meaning of a metaphor (290). The dynamic aspects of a reader's response to a metaphor connects its distinctive concepts according to the diverse ideologies that they have imbibed through time. In a given context, the focal word/vehicle "obtains a *new* meaning, which is *not* quite its meaning in literal uses, not quite the meaning which any literary substitute would have. The new context imposes *extension* of meaning upon the focal word" (Black 286); also, the new implications thus constructed by the reader will be determined by the pattern of implications associated with literal uses of the vehicle and tenor. These patterns and assumed literal usages function according to what Black calls "the system of associated commonplaces" (287). In the process of meaning interaction and transference, Black observes, some of the associated commonplaces also suffer metaphorical change of meaning, most of which can be described as "*extensions* of meaning" (289) as they do not involve perceived connections between the two conceptual systems.

Most attributes of the interaction theory of metaphors are relevant to the study of the visual metaphors that abound in graphic pathographies. The novel meanings that emerge during metaphor comprehension are of immense significance in expressing intangible and intimate psychological experiences that cannot be conveyed in either of the conceptual systems (of the vehicle and tenor) but necessarily require metaphorical interactions. Further, in a medium that involves an active reader in the process of meaning making through comics closure, the metaphorical processes converge with those aspects of comics reading where the reader creates meaning in a context-oriented interaction with images from diverse conceptual systems.

### *Conceptual Metaphor Theory (CMT)*

Recent research on metaphor has attempted to dismantle the presumptions regarding metaphor as a linguistic tool by exploring and demonstrating its cognitive dimensions. The preliminary analysis of metaphors as an inherent part of conceptual system was undertaken by George Lakoff and Mark Johnson in *Metaphors We Live By* (1980). They proposed that "metaphor is pervasive in everyday life, not just in language but in thought and action" (3), and that "our ordinary conceptual system, in terms of which we both think and act, is fundamentally metaphorical in nature" (3). Thus, redeeming metaphors from its conception as a matter of language, these cognitive theorists argued that they are a significant tool by means of which reality is conceptualised, thereby impacting the behaviours and actions of the users of language. In contrast to comparison and transference theories that regard metaphors as extraordinary and ornamental, CMT foregrounds the use of metaphors in everyday language. Deploying instances from everyday language, Lakoff and Johnson demonstrate how metaphorical concepts are realised in 'natural' speech. For instance, the following expressions from colloquial language are based on the conceptual metaphor ARGUMENT IS WAR:

> Your claims are *indefensible*.
> He *attacked every weak point* in my argument.
> His criticisms were *right on target*.
> I *demolished* his argument.
> He *shot down* all my arguments.

(4)

As evinced by the italicised words drawn from the conceptual category of war in the above example, Lakoff and Johnson argue that more than mere comparison, "[t]he essence of metaphor is understanding and experiencing one kind of thing in terms of another" (5). For instance, as the abovementioned sentences expose how most part of the ordinary arguments are partially structured by the concept of war (4), one could argue that the concept, activity, and language of war is metaphorically structured. Although Lakoff and Johnson attempt to propose the universality of this conceptual structure in most everyday argumentative speech, they also hint at the cultural differences that could engender diverse formulations of metaphorical structuring. In a culture where arguments lack any sense of attack or defence, gaining or losing, and instead are viewed as a dance, the objective would be to present oneself in a balanced and pleasing way (5). In other words, recognition of distinct conceptual structures in terms of discourse formation resolves the cultural conflict and its consequent influence on cognitive metaphorical structures.

## Metaphors and Contexts

According to CMT, the mapping of two distinct conceptual domains (source to the target) takes place not by comparison but based on the correlation of the user's experience in the two domains of thought and his/her ability to structure one abstract concept in terms of another.

Orientational metaphors, as Lakoff and Johnson would call them, foreground spatialisation of physical and cultural experience in their use. For instance, the following statements are grounded on the conceptual metaphor HAPPY IS UP; SAD IS DOWN, as drooping posture is typically associated with sadness and depression and erect posture with a positive emotional state:

> I'm feeling *down*.
> That *boosted* my interest.
> I *fell* into a depression.
> My spirits *sank*.

However, by giving examples of conceptual categories that betray clear conflict between mainstream and marginal cultural values, CMT theorists declare any attempt to link metaphorical expressions to a standard account of meaning as futile. Experiential gestalts—structured wholes within recurrent human experiences—that characterise the conceptual categories of a metaphor themselves are not always universal but could also vary from culture to culture (Lakoff and Johnson 117). Further, these gestalts are products of interactions with one's physical environment, as well as with other people within one's culture. Taking cues from this argument, El Refaie proposes that basic sensorimotor experiences are deeply imbued with socio-cultural meanings, in that bodily experiences become not just the source, but also the target of metaphorical mappings. Departing from most metaphor theorists, who tend to operate under static and deterministic notions of culture and society, El Refaie argues: "the body does not constitute a prediscursive, material reality; rather, it ... is constantly being constructed and reconstructed on the basis of social and cultural assumptions about class, gender, sex, race, ethnicity, age, health, and beauty" ("Appearances" 111). El Refaie, based on Pritzker's notion, argues for the perception of cultural models as a rich resource that individuals can exploit in order to create meaningful stories of their bodily experiences.

Delineating the socio-cultural models of analysing visual metaphors, in "Understanding Visual Metaphor: The Example of Newspaper Cartoons," El Refaie proposes a context-dependent method. She argues that even 'conventionality,' which is foregrounded in the cognitive model, is an elusive concept, thereby emphasising the significance of specific socio-cultural contexts in analysing conceptual metaphors:

> [T]he degree to which the connections between two concepts strikes us as literal or metaphorical does not depend on any

objective distance between the two but rather on how deeply the connection is 'entrenched' in our conceptual system, in other words, on how conventional it is. In fact, conventionality is also rather an elusive concept, which cannot be determined once and for all but depends on the specific discourse context.

(82)

While the tenor and vehicle of the metaphor are explicitly stated in the verbal mode, in a visual metaphor, an abstract entity cannot be depicted without the mediation of symbols or metaphors. Even in the absence of the tenor, Forceville observes that context assumes a pertinent role in determining the meaning of a verbo-visual metaphor (qtd. in El Refaie, "Understanding" 85). In distinguishing pictorial context, linguistic context, and world knowledge, Forceville uses Barthes's theory of text-image relations. Accordingly, the linguistic message is functionally referred to as 'anchorage,' as images by nature are 'polysemous' in a floating chain of signifieds (Barthes 39). However, in reading the verbo-visual metaphors, El Refaie prefers the theory proposed by Kress and van Leeuwen to Barthes's "unidirectional concept of anchorage" ("Understanding" 86) which grants preference to the verbal message over the visual. Kress and van Leeuwen, on the other hand, propose a mutual influence between the distinct semiotic modes and assume that verbal and visual meanings "intermesh and interact at all times" (40). Taking these cues, El Refaie analyses the verbo-visual metaphors in newspaper cartoons based on the verbal context (located in close proximity to the image), and the broader discourse context (all other items of text on a newspaper page), which Forceville calls "world knowledge" (qtd. in El Refaie, "Understanding" 86). El Refaie thus lays bare the immense range of possible interpretations of a verbo-visual metaphor, as their context-dependencies are more implicit than explicit. Accordingly, she goes on to argue that "the depiction of an abstract entity in the visual mode is utterly impossible without the mediation of metaphors" (91).

Noel Carroll differentiates the visual metaphor from the verbal metaphor through what he refers to as 'homospatiality,' or, in other words, a fusion of ideas within the same space (190). In the visual metaphor, he argues, two "discrete elements coexist in the same space, ... and call ... to mind different concepts or categories" (191, 193). Another element of the visual metaphor, for Carroll, is that the image at hand must be 'physically noncompossible,' which implies that the viewer should perceive those elements in the same space, not as "a representation of a physically possible state of affairs, but as an opportunity to regard one of the categories as providing a source for apprehending something about the other category" (199). As such, Carroll establishes the nature of visual metaphor as the fusion of two distinct images (or ideas) that should not be interpreted distinctly on their own. Carroll states that "in determining whether the elements in an array are physically noncompossible, ... we need to consider the context in which the image is presented and the intentions of the image-maker in presenting it" (208). In a similar vein, Charles Forceville, who has published at length about pictorial metaphor, understands it as a phenomenon in which a visual replacement of expectations occurs (El Refaie, "Understanding" 80).

Further, based on Lakoff and Johnson's argument about metaphor as a conceptual phenomenon, El Refaie argues that "it must be expressible in many different modes, not just language" ("Analysing" 148). In such a context, the metaphors used in graphic memoirs/autobiographical comics gain import, as most of the metaphors deployed in them reveal an acute engagement with the visualisation of internal bodily processes that are otherwise inaccessible.

## Multimodal Metaphors and Illness Depiction

The study of metaphors in non-linguistic domains has led to the analysis of entities that are more depictable (source domain) to describe those that are less depictable (target domain). This scholarship, which combines two or more modalities of human expression, has been labelled as the study of multimodal metaphors. As multimodal metaphors operate by combining images and text, and thereby involve characteristics like spatial configuration, size, clarity, and colour, Forceville and Eduardo argue that they are "more noticeable in visual discourses than in verbal ones" (13). Although metaphors are generally classified into verbal, visual, and verbo-visual, Forceville (2007, 2009) distinguishes between five categories of 'pictorial metaphors':

- *Hybrid metaphor*: In hybrid metaphors, both the source and target are partially pictured and joined together into one figure that is perceived as a single, unified object. Carroll's (1994) examples of fusion and homospatiality fall under this category.
- *Pictorial simile*: Pictorial similes are characterised by both the source and target being visually depicted in their entirety as two separate figures, but in a way that emphasises their similarity.
- *Contextual metaphor*: In contextual metaphors, only the source or the target is depicted, in a context where normally something else would be expected; the replacement of the anticipated element encourages viewers to interpret one thing in terms of another.

- *Integrated metaphor*: In this type of metaphor, "[a] phenomenon that is experienced as a unified object or gestalt is represented in its entirety in such a manner that it resembles another object or gestalt even without contextual cues" (Forceville 18).
- *Verbo-pictorial metaphors*: Either the source or the target is not pictured but is implied instead by the verbal message.

Among these categories, only 'verbo-pictorial metaphors' are multimodal, as they draw on both the visual and the verbal modes. As such, these metaphors are used in the comics medium, which performs meaning through an interplay of both word and image. For instance, in a verbo-pictorial metaphor used by Ellen Forney in her graphic memoir, *Marbles*, the source (a bipolar patient at varied angles on a carousel) is conveyed both visually (excited and depressed gestures of the patient) and verbally (handwritten text), while the target (stages of bipolar condition) is not represented exclusively in the image and thus depends heavily upon verbal cues (medical registers of bipolarity). As a composite medium, comics constantly reconciles and mediates the verbal and visual codes allowing the representation of intricate realities and lived experiences that often escape verbal presentation. Particularly, the conceptual metaphors deployed in comics serve "to conceptualize the world, define notions of reality and construct subjectivity" (Lupton 59). In a way, these metaphors are inevitable for narrating illness experiences, in that they concretise and define abstract and chaotic realms of the psyche. Given such affordances, it is not surprising that Williams regards metaphor as a pivotal feature of comics. Metaphors at once crystallises affective states and mental intricacies for which no apposite verbal language exists. To quote Williams, "the multilayered perceptual representations of graphic narrative [constituted through metaphors] are well suited to the portrayal of mental health problems" (78). In their endeavour to embody experiences and to forge meaningful accounts of their own illnesses, graphic memoirists often exploit metaphors grounded on bodily actions and sensory perceptions. Although metaphors and other rhetorical tropes cannot completely recreate an irreducible subjective experience, they serve in approximating the author's idiosyncratic emotions (Huyssen 133; Whitlock 977). For instance, Matthew Johnstone's graphic memoir, *I Had a Black Dog*, depicts a series of fantastic incidents where the black dog, which embodies Johnstone's depression, haunts and consumes his everyday life. The author's feelings of inadequacy and diffidence caused by depression are reproduced through the metaphor of a black dog which varies in size/shape according to the author's varied phases of depression (Johnstone).

In close-reading visual metaphors deployed in graphic memoirs of mental illness, we will follow the "tripartite taxonomy of visual metaphor" (81) proposed by El Refaie in her seminal work, *Visual Metaphor and Embodiment in Graphic Illness Narratives*. As such, visual metaphor types are classified into pictorial, spatial, and stylistic metaphors. Forceville's categories of metaphors mentioned above are grouped under pictorial metaphors. When metaphorical meanings emerge from "correlations between the experience of our bodies in space and more abstract concepts," El Refaie categorises it as spatial metaphor (*Visual Metaphor* 117). Within this category, when spatial relations in the storyworld evoke metaphorical meanings, they constitute diegetic spatial metaphors. When spatial relations of verbal or visual elements on the page or double-page spread evoke metaphorical meanings, they constitute compositional spatial metaphor. When the style of pictures, words, abstract visual elements like pictorial runes or the materiality of the book constitutes the source domain of a metaphorical mapping, they are called stylistic metaphors. Within this category, the basic visual attributes that suggest abstract meanings are grouped as isomorphic stylistic metaphors, and other higher-order features of style (such as modes of production and digital techniques) that evoke metaphorical meaning are grouped as indexical stylistic metaphors (117).

Combining the arguments of conceptual metaphor theorists with multimodality, it can be observed that most of the metaphors under discussion draws on "concrete, clearly structured experiences of our bodily actions and perceptions as a way to understand abstract, non-physical domains such as mental states, emotions and social relations" (El Refaie, "Analysing" 153). As such, representation of subjective and abstract experiences like chronic pain and illness necessitates the use of metaphors. Elena Semino has observed that both "the clinical and the social scientific literature on pain" has recognised sufferers' frequent employment of figurative language in expressing their pain experiences (207). Distinct from biomedical repertoires of disease representations, figurative language, specifically metaphors, abound in autobiographical narratives on illness experience. These narratives of illness experience, specifically graphic pathographies, are considered significant for this study, as they offer a unique language and terms of representation in which the totality of patienthood and illness experience can be reflected upon, integrated into the life of the sufferer, and shared with others. Along with the aforementioned graphic narratives chosen for this study, several non-Anglo-American graphic narratives such as David B's *Epileptic* (*L'Ascension du haut mal*) (1996), David Ramírez's *COnviVIenDo 19 days* (2020), and several Japanese "medical manga" (Nakagaki) also make use of verbo-visual metaphors in their delineation of illness experience. Our recent article on the COVID-19 comics and metaphors titled "Comics in the Time of a Pan(dem)ic: COVID-19, Graphic Medicine, and Metaphors," for instance, explores the wide use of metaphorical expressions to convey the pandemic condition (Saji et al. 152). These narratives, in other words, provide a "pedagogy of expressive possibility" (Frank 182). Inspired by Elaine Scarry, David Biro in his *Language of Pain* qualifies metaphors with a specific clinical value which "has the power to alleviate pain" (145). Describing pain as a metaphoric 'black hole' into which language disappears, Biro underlines his major theoretical argument that both expression and understanding of pain are dependent on metaphors: "[w]e don't have a way of understanding and talking about pain without metaphors," he affirms. "If we are to speak at all, we must use metaphors" (77).

However, metaphors in the context of illness have been contested since Susan Sontag's *Illness as Metaphor*. Sontag argues that "the most truthful way of regarding illness—and the healthiest way of being ill—is one most purified of, most resistant to, metaphoric thinking" (3). Sontag examines metaphors of illness that infiltrate the conceptualisation of disease as "evil, invincible predator" (7). She traces several figurative uses of diseases as a metaphor for monstrosity and destructiveness in nineteenth-century literature. Especially in literary discussions and representations of diseases like cancer and TB, the predominant metaphor used was that of war and invasion; to quote Sontag, "[i]n TB, the person is 'consumed,' burned up. In cancer, the patient is 'invaded' by alien cells" (14). In the revised edition of Sontag's book, she clarifies how military metaphors "contribute to the stigmatizing of certain illnesses and by extension, of those who are ill" (97). Quite interestingly, originally, the metaphors of TB signified romantic ideals of beauty and higher social status. In course of time, the metaphors associated with tuberculosis and insanity started to have parallels of a psychic voyage, which was an extension of the romantic idea of a journey. From these cues, it can be perceived that metaphors evolve through social and cultural prejudices about illness. At the same time, this pattern underscores the pervading *presence* of metaphors in expressions/representations of illness experiences. Sontag herself begins *Illness as Metaphor* with the conceptual metaphorical mapping of illness to journey:

> everyone who is born holds a dual citizenship, in the kingdom of the well and in the kingdom of the sick. Although we all prefer to

use only the good passport, sooner or later each of us is obliged, at
least for a spell, to identify ourselves as citizens of that other place.
(3)

Though critical of the use of metaphors in the first edition of *Illness
as Metaphor*, the above statement undergirds inevitability of metaphors in everyday language and discourses on healthcare. However,
Sontag clarified her position regarding her resistance to metaphorical
representations of illness in the related 1988 work *AIDS and its Metaphors*. She elucidates her arguments against the use of metaphors of
illness in the specific case of war metaphors that tend to stigmatise patients and deprive them of effective means of coping with their illness.

Despite such criticisms, the growing research in metaphorical representations of illness experience no longer categorise metaphor as a
'figure of speech' but as a 'figure of thought.' As Frank observes, "a
metaphor is no longer a trope, in the sense of twisting language. Instead, reality is what is twisted, and language is a straightening out
process" (193).

## Why Metaphors?

The use of figurative language/rhetorical devices is critical in reconstructing the life-world of the patient, which is impaired by the onset
of illness. As Frank remarks, metaphors bridge the gap between the
reality of the sufferer and that of the healthy reader:

> [w]hen the 'hard reality' of metaphorical, figurative, and evoc-
> ative expressions found in illness narratives meet with the hard
> reality of non-depressed and healthy-bodied readers, a rhetorical
> situation is created in the 'communication between simultaneous
> differences.'
>
> (qtd. in Martinez 18)

Such negotiations of the differences between the autobiographical
subject and the reader not only facilitate a lucid translation of the author's altered reality engendered by illness but also formulate ways of
recovering the author's lost sense of identity through shared feelings.
Shaped by one's perceptions and cultural affinities with others, metaphor thus becomes an inevitable rhetorical device to form concepts
about self and to describe personal experiences to others.

The use of metaphors is thus inevitable to any expressions of illness
experiences. Frank attests to the inevitability of using metaphors in

illness narratives and critiques the approach of biomedicine which is grounded on symptoms:

> [M]etaphor is already such an essential part of people's expression. Pain and illness call for expanding metaphoric repertoires, and first-person narratives often tell regrettable tales of institutional medicine stultifying metaphorical capacity instead of nurturing it, thus creating barriers to communication and self-understanding.
>
> (186)

Frank also argues that several autopathographies "offer a language—terms of representation—in which disease, pain, and the often surreal impositions of treatment can be reflected upon, integrated into the life of the sufferer, and shared with others" through metaphors (182).

In the context of narrating mental illness experiences, the use of metaphors has been recognised as an effective tool in psychotherapy (Barlow et al. 212). Several such studies (Mould et al. 282; Sayce 132) have found that fragmented experiences of self are inherent to psychotic disorders and that reconstructing one's sense of self is an integral part of recovery process. However, owing to the complexities of articulating the experience of mental illness, authors often rely on the use of conventional/familiar metaphors. Accordingly, metaphors can act as a bridge between the patient's narrative and the physician's clinical knowledge about mental illness. For instance, metaphors of illness that are rooted in specific cultural contexts and those that foreground spatialisation of physical experience reveal unvocalised psychic turmoil. In such contexts, if physicians are trained in recognising and valuing metaphors as part of comprehending the patient's narrative through health humanities/graphic medicine in medical curriculum, productive doctor-patient dynamics ensues. As Charon proposes, in most clinical encounters, the physician had to follow "the patient's narrative thread, identify the metaphors or images used in the telling, tolerate ambiguity and uncertainty as the story unfolded, identify the unspoken subtexts, and hear one story in light of others told by this teller" (4). Adherence to an impersonal symptom checklist like the *Diagnostic and Statistical Manual of Mental Disorders* (DSM) for treating the mentally ill, on the contrary, hinders the physician/psychiatrist from engaging in a productive discussion of the patient's personal experiences (Andreasen 111).

As memoirs on mental illness depict extra-verbal realities, each author faces a rhetorical challenge as these representations may contradict socially constructed rhetorical resources (Martinez 20). The figurative and metaphorical ways in which each author narrates these extra-verbal rhetorical challenges thus perform as a critique of the extant meanings of cultural practices in the mode of their illness condition. Moreover, it cannot be assumed that memoirs on mental illness that deploy figurative techniques easily convey the intricacies of the illness experience to the reader as there is no fixed notion of selfhood which anyone can identify with. Instead, narrative depictions of disordered experiences communicate a distinct self with whom a reader might encounter in the course of reading the particular memoir. As Martinez remarks, "the figurative narrative passages about disordered realties continually interpose a distance between normative understandings and disordered experiences. This generates a symbolic division that catalyze non-depressed audiences to interpretatively bridge the gap" through juxtaposition of their own normative reality alongside the personal experiences of the authors (190). In this context, the fragmentary nature of the comics medium along with its paralinguistic elements such as panel shapes, gutter spaces, or emanatas aids the author to highlight her own uncertainty and the fragmentary nature of her experience in an immediate fashion.

El Refaie and Semino argue that metaphors enable us to comprehend complex and abstract aspects of reality in more concrete, familiar, and easily imaginable terms. Therefore, in the context of mental illness, metaphors help artists to effectively encapsulate their psychic turmoils in vivid details which often escapes literal expressions. Recognising the significance of metaphorical expressions of mental illness, a recent initiative by Cardiff University, "DrawingOut Invisible Diseases," encourages people with mental illness to express themselves through visual metaphors through their website www.drawingout.org. The web gallery of drawings by patients serve as an online platform where a community of sufferers "share their thoughts and feelings about their condition" ("DrawingOut"). While metaphors serve social functions in persuading, entertaining, and establishing intimacy between the author and the reader, they could also function as an ideological weapon in its process of mapping structure from a source domain to a target domain, thereby foregrounding specific aspects of a concept while hiding others. Such power relations engendered by the use of specific metaphors and complementary narrative strategies, especially in the context of mental illness, will be discussed in detail in the next chapter.

## Conclusion

Metaphors provide an alternative to the claims that objectivity is the only choice in perceiving the truth about an experience. Labelled as "imaginative rationality" (Lakoff and Johnson 193), metaphors unite reason with imagination and validate an experientialist account of perception and comprehension of complex emotions and abstract feelings. As Bleakley reminds, metaphors acknowledge and transform "the ordinary into the extraordinary through transposition, gaining deeper meanings or more effective traction" (208). The context-based experiential approach to visual metaphors further bridges the gap between objectivist and subjectivist assumptions about impartial expressions and representations of truth about mental illness experiences. Such an approach enables readers/listeners and analysts of metaphors to perceive truth as relative to one's conceptual system, which is in a constant state of flux and evolution, shaped by human experiences.

## Reference List

Abrams, M. H. *A Glossary of Literary Terms*. 7th ed., Heinle and Heinle, 1999.

Andreasen, Nancy C. "DSM and the Death of Phenomenology in America: An Example of Unintended Consequences." *Schizophrenia Bulletin*, vol. 33, no. 1, 2007, pp. 108–112.

Barlow, Jack M., et al. "Insight and Figurative Language in Psychotherapy." *Psychotherapy: Theory, Research & Practice*, vol. 14, no. 3, 1977, pp. 212–222.

Barthes, Roland. *Image-Music-Text*. Translated by Stephen Heath. Fontana, 1977.

Biro, David. *Language of Pain: Finding Words, Compassion, and Relief*. Norton, 2010.

Black, Max. "Metaphor." *Proceedings of the Aristotelian Society*, vol. 55, no. 1, 1955, pp. 273–294.

Bleakley, Alan. *Thinking with Metaphors in Medicine: The State of the Art*. Routledge, 2017.

Cacciari, Cristina. "Why Do We Speak Metaphorically: Reflections on the Functions of Metaphor in Discourse and Reasoning." *Figurative Language and Thought*, edited by Albert N. Katz et al., Oxford UP, 1998, pp. 119–157.

Carroll, Noel. "Visual Metaphor." *Aspects of Metaphor*, edited by Jaako Hintikka, Springer and Business Media, 1994, pp. 189–218.

Charon, Rita. *Narrative Medicine: Honoring the Stories of Illness*. Oxford UP, 2006.

"DrawingOut Invisible Disease." DrawingOut, https://drawingout.org/about/.

El Refaie, Elisabeth. "Analysing Metaphors in Multimodal Texts." *The Routledge Handbook of Metaphor and Language*, edited by Elena Semino and Zsófia Demjén, Routledge, 2017, pp. 148–162.

———. "Appearances and Dis/Dys-appearances: A Dynamic View of Embodiment in Conceptual Metaphor Theory." *Metaphor and the Social World*, vol. 4, no. 1, 2014, pp. 109–125.

———. "Understanding Visual Metaphor: The Example of Newspaper Cartoons." *Visual Communication*, vol. 2, no. 75, 2003, pp. 75–95.

———. *Visual Metaphor and Embodiment in Graphic Illness Narratives*. Oxford UP, 2019.

Forceville, Charles. "Multimodal Metaphor in Ten Dutch TV Commercials." *Public Journal of Semiotics*, vol. 1, 2007, pp. 19–51.

———, and Urios-Aparisi Eduardo, editors. *Multimodal Metaphor*. Mouton de Gruyter, 2009.

Frank, Arthur. "Metaphors of Pain." *Literature and Medicine*, vol. 29, no. 1, 2011, pp. 182–196.

Halliwell, Stephen. *The Poetics of Aristotle: Translation and Commentary*. Duckworth, 1987.

Huyssen, Andreas. *Present Pasts: Urban Palimpsests and the Politics of Memory*. Stanford UP, 2003.

Isenberg, Arnold. "On Defining Metaphor." *Journal of Philosophy*, vol. 60, no. 21, 1963, pp. 609–622.

Johnstone, Matthew. *I Had a Black Dog: His Name Was Depression*. Robinson, 2007.

Kirby, John T. "Aristotle on Metaphor." *American Journal of Philology*, vol. 118, no. 4, 1997, pp. 517–554.

Kress, Gunther, and Theo van Leeuwen. *Reading Images: The Grammar of Visual Design*. Routledge, 1996.

Lakoff, George, and Mark Johnson. *Metaphors We Live By: With a New Afterword*. The U of Chicago P, 2003.

Lupton, Deborah. *Medicine as Culture: Illness, Disease and the Body in Western Societies*. Sage, 2003.

Martinez, Jermaine. "Rhetorical Dimensions of 20th Century Depression Memoirs: Sylvia Plath's The Bell Jar, William Styron's Darkness Visible, & Kay Redfield Jamison's An Unquiet Mind." U of Illinois at Urbana-Champaign, 2016. PhD Dissertation.

Mould, Tracy J., et al. "The Use of Metaphor for Understanding and Managing Psychotic Experiences: A Systematic Review." *Journal of Mental Health*, vol. 19, no. 3, 2010, pp. 282–293.

Nakagaki, Kotaro. "Development of 'Medical Manga' in Overseas Manga." *Medical Manga*, 19 May 2021, https://graphicmedicine.jp/medical-manga/column12/.

Nöth, Winfried. *Handbook of Semiotics*. Indiana UP, 1995.

Richards, I. A. *The Philosophy of Rhetoric*. Oxford UP, 1936.

Saji, Sweetha, et al. "Comics in the Time of a Pan(dem)ic: COVID-19, Graphic Medicine, and Metaphors." *Perspectives in Biology and Medicine*, vol. 64, no. 1, winter 2021, pp. 136–154.

Sayce, Liz. *From Psychiatric Patient to Citizen: Overcoming Discrimination and Social Exclusion*. Macmillan, 2000.

Semino, Elena. "Descriptions of Pain, Metaphor, and Embodied Simulation." *Metaphor and Symbol*, vol. 25, no. 4, 2010, pp. 205–226.

Sontag, Susan. *Illness as Metaphor: AIDS and Its Metaphors.* Penguin, 1991.

Whitlock, Gillian. "Autographics: The Seeing "I" of the Comics." *Mfs Modern Fiction Studies*, vol. 52, no. 4, 2006, pp. 965–979.

Williams, Ian. "Graphic Medicine: The Portrayal of Illness in Underground and Autobiographical Comics." *Medicine, Health and the Arts: Approaches to the Medical Humanities*, edited by Victoria Bates et al., Routledge, 2014, pp. 64–84.

# 3  Mental Illness and the Politics of Representation

## Introduction

Representation, primarily understood as 'presence' or 'appearance' with an implied visual component, is a critical concept in the cultural milieu. Conceived as "clear images, material reproductions, performances and simulations" (Baldonado), representations propagate through various media: films, television, photographs, advertisements, and other forms of popular culture. In the introduction to *Picture Theory*, W. J. T. Mitchell elaborates the function of representation thus: "representation (in memory, in verbal descriptions, in images) not only 'mediates' our knowledge (of slavery and of many other things), but obstructs, fragments, and negates that knowledge" (188). In other words, representation does not only channel the knowledge we consume, it also constructs knowledge. Second, Mitchell resists the notion of representations as particular kinds of objects. Instead, he treats them "as relationship, as process, as the relay mechanism in exchanges of power, value, and publicity" (420). Mitchell's model proposes an approach to representation with an eye toward the relationships and processes through which representations are produced, valued, and exchanged. As such, Andrew Edgar and Peter Sedgwick in *Key Concepts in Cultural Theory* characterise 'representation' as "the 'presentation' or construction of identity [which] may be closely allied to questions of ideology and power, and to the forms of discourse implicated in the procedures whereby such images are created" (225). In a similar vein, Ella Shohat poses some fundamental questions on the nature of representations and the ideologies that frame them:

> [e]ach filmic or academic utterance must be analyzed not only in terms of who represents but also in terms of who is being

DOI: 10.4324/9781003214229-4

represented, for what purpose, at which historical moment, from which location, using which strategies, and in what tone of address.

(173)

Shohat's questions on the ideological framework that determines the nature of representations also lay bare the politics of representation. Rather than perceiving representations as "harmless likenesses" (Baldonado), they must be analysed for the ways in which they impact perceptions. Stuart Hall addresses the politics of representation in *Representation: Cultural Representations and Signifying Practices*, in that he approaches representation as the medium or channel through which production of meaning happens. He assumes that objects or people do not have stable, true meanings, but rather that the meanings are produced by participants in a culture, who have the power to signify something (3). Clearly, for Hall, representation involves understanding how language and systems of knowledge production work together to produce and circulate meanings. Representation becomes the process or channel through which these meanings are both created and reified.

As such, abuse of the power of representation can be clearly observed in several socio-cultural phenomena especially in the context of AIDS in the 1980s and slavery during colonialism. Nancy L Roth and Katy Hogan in *Gendered Epidemic: Representations of Women in the Age of AIDS* explore the representations of AIDS in mainstream and medical discourse along these lines. As such, they cite several mainstream media and medical news reports which represent AIDS as "a new mystery disease plaguing gay men"; "epidemic of immune deficiency"; and the plight of "hemophiliacs and infants, the 'innocent victims' of the epidemic" (115). They underline the role of perspective or framing in the production of negative representations of illness based on 'media frames' theory of Hall. In so doing, they seek to explain how "hegemonic discourse selects, orders, or excludes certain versions of reality in its effort to organize the world according to its own purposes" (Roth and Hogan 136).

Paula A. Treichler questions the correspondence that is presumed to exist between "the representation of [AIDS] virus and its reality" by examining the features of the culture that determine the form in which reality is constructed and the "role of language in articulation and popularizing a particular construction" (151). Treichler observes that by 1986, the major newsmagazines in the US were running the cover stories on "the grave danger that AIDS posed to heterosexuals" (18).

As such, representations of AIDS as a 'gay disease' in news magazines, televisions, and posters in a way not only protect "sexual practices of heterosexuality but also heterosexuality's ideological superiority" (22–23). These ideological tools were operated in subtle ways of visual representations of AIDS in popular magazines. The severity of the epidemic was heightened by a shift from images of gay men with their arms entwined and aloof gay man in a backlit apartment to nuclear families, 'innocent victims,' and middle-American patriots who were at 'risk.' For instance, the July 1985 issue of *Life* magazine contributed a distinct iconography of the epidemic that suggests this shift. As Treichler observes,

> In living color, photographs of people with AIDS stared out at the reader: an African-American soldier in uniform, saluting; the Burks, a white all-American nuclear family (father, mother, daughter, baby-son); and an attractive young blonde woman. In bold red letters, the cover warned that "NOW NO ONE IS SAFE FROM AIDS." ... The cover illustration made visual the magazine's position: "AIDS is a problem for all." An effort was made, in other words, to articulate AIDS to important elements of a liberal democracy—we're all equal, we're in this together, we are family—and to freight the "faces of AIDS" on the cover.
>
> (75–76)

Representations thus act as ideological tools of interpretation that control perceptions about the marginalised who do not hold power over their own representations. Stereotyped representations of Africans served as ideological tools supporting colonialism and slavery. Moreover, they served to justify racial difference and segregation, and protected the freedom that white supremacists enjoyed. European representations of Africa and its people as 'dark,' 'savage,' and 'violent' perpetuated a perverse opposite to its 'civilised' life thereby maintaining European superiority as self-evident. Edward Said, in his analysis of textual representations of the Orient in *Orientalism*, proposes that representations cannot be realistic:

> In any instance of at least written language, there is no such thing as a delivered presence, but a *re-presence*, or a representation. The value, efficacy, strength, apparent veracity of a written statement about the Orient therefore relies very little, and cannot instrumentally depend, on the Orient as such. On the contrary, the written statement is a presence to the reader by virtue of its having

excluded, displaced, made supererogatory any such *real thing* as "the Orient."

(88)

Said dispels the objectivity claimed by European representations of Africa as constructed images interspersed with clear ideological content.

Similarly, representations of mental illness perform a pivotal role in framing perceptions about the mentally ill. These representations are not devoid of meaning and hence influence and shape public perceptions about the illness. Sensationalised and distorted images of the mentally ill, for instance, lead to stereotyping of mental illness as a disease of deviance and abnormality contributing to the stigma that negatively impacts those who experience the travails of the illness. Ato Quayson in "Aesthetic Nervousness" argues that representations of disability/illness are not mere replicas of a stable and inert outside reality, and thus, the ethical dimensions of representing illness cannot be subsumed under mere aesthetic dimensions. Accordingly, he argues that "the representation of disability oscillates uneasily between the aesthetic and the ethical domains" and that the disability representation from the perspective of the disabled is crucially distinct "from the normative position of the nondisabled" (205). Worse still, scientific accounts of mental illness are also not productively equipped to dismantle misconceptions; instead, they concentrate on symptoms over the lived experience of the patients as individuals. As Gilman rightly comments on the negative visualisations of madness in medicine and popular art in *Seeing the Insane*, our understanding of the mentally ill is predicated on "the continued presence in society of older images of the insane, images that overtly or covertly color our concept and serve to categorize them upon first glance" (iii). As these mediations of madness can be copied or reproduced, their accessibility increases on a mass level and gradually leading to its legitimisation.

This chapter aims to analyse how mental illness is perceived, represented, and treated in popular culture and medical discourses. In so doing, this chapter lays bare the ideologies and the symbolic codes that undergird these representations and the consequent stigma confronted by the mentally ill. Although 'popular culture' is interpreted as "the culture that appeals to, or that is most comprehensible by, the general public," the term is used frequently "either to identify a form of culture that is opposed to another form, or as a synonym or complement to that other form" (Edgar and Sedgwick 190–191). As such, popular culture may refer either to "individual artefacts (often treated as texts) such as a popular song or a television programme, or to a group's lifestyle (and thus to the pattern of artefacts, practices and understandings that serve to establish the group's distinctive identity)" (191). Taking these cues, this chapter close-reads popular representations of mental illness in movies, newspapers, advertisements, comics, and paintings and the articulation of stereotyped images of the mentally ill in medical discourse which externalise madness in distorted physiognomic features. In so doing, this chapter attempts to expose the negative implications of these representations on the personal and social lives of the mentally ill.

## Defining Mental Illness

Psychiatry, one of the oldest of the medical specialities in the treatment of the mentally ill, grew into prominence by the dawn of modern science and during the Enlightenment (Lewis 65). Grounded on scientific postulates, psychiatry followed the method of investigation with clear and detailed case descriptions and objectives. However, the influence of the Enlightenment ideals which emphasised the value of dignity and individuality of the human being led to the inclusion of a variety of psychotherapeutic techniques personalising the care to the individual's needs. In such an amalgamation of the benefits of modern science with the philosophy of the Enlightenment, psychiatry gained a moral grounding that it strived to maintain. By the rise of Freudian psychoanalysis as an alternative approach to mentalscapes in the mid-twentieth century, psychiatry was challenged with its declining emphasis on observable signs and symptoms. Psychoanalysis in general focussed on intrapsychic conflicts over diagnosis and classifications. As a response to this critical turn, the American Psychiatric Association (APA) codified various psychiatric disorders in the *Diagnostic and Statistical Manual of Mental Disorders* (DSM). Although the DSM existed prior to the rise of psychoanalysis, it was in 1980 that the APA initiated the need for a definition of mental disorders in the third edition of the DSM. Aimed at maximum reliability and validity, DSM-III and its revised fourth edition gradually became "universally and uncritically accepted as the ultimate authority on psychopathology and diagnosis" (Andreasen 111). Mental illness as given in the DSM refers to the spectrum of cognition, emotions, and behaviours that interfere with interpersonal relationships as well as familial and societal functions (Johnstone, "Stigma" 203). As such, the DSM is still commonly recognised the 'psychiatric bible.'

However, this codification, aimed at defending psychiatry's scientific status, had a dehumanising impact. In being reduced to mere check-lists, clinicians who frequent the DSM as a toolkit fail to approach patients as individuals (Pearce 515). The immediate requirement of a codified data was fulfilled at the cost of comprehensive descriptions that addressed patient needs. Moreover, certain categories of mental disorders listed in the DSM were not tested for validity. Adding to this crisis, as Horgan remarks, unlike "definitions of ischemic heart disease, lymphoma, or AIDS, the DSM diagnoses are based on a consensus about clusters of clinical symptoms, not any objective laboratory measure." Moreover, an overview of the categories of mental disorders that made into the DSM reveals false prejudices that catered to dehumanising attitudes towards the marginal groups in society. For instance, in the 1850s, a physician called Samuel Cartwright coined a term, 'drapetomania' referring to the psychological condition that caused black slaves to run away (Myers). Similarly, homosexuality was listed as a 'sociopathic personality disorder' in the DSM until 1973. Apart from psychologists and psychiatrists, the DSM was widely used in various social firms like insurance companies, courts, prisons, and other social services agencies in determining those eligible for special services and reimbursements. As such, blind approval of the DSM's categories and criteria was carefully reconsidered.

In the subsequent editions of the DSM, alternative perspectives from social, cultural, political dimensions were regarded as significant prerequisites accompanying the characteristic symptoms of a particular diagnosis. These additional aspects of diagnosis were aimed at developing clinicians' sensitivity to the patients' resilience and personal experiences over their perceived deficits. The latest edition of the DSM (DSM-5) has created a common lexicon used by psychiatrists and mental healthcare providers in the diagnosis of mental disorders. Evolving as a comprehensive guide to understanding the nuances of living with and perceiving mental disorders, the DSM-5 takes into account both clinical and cultural symptoms in determining the diagnosis. As such, the manual provides a list of factors and interview questions in terms of race, ethnicity, language, religion, social customs, geographical origins, etc., in reckoning a patient's illness experience. Further, it also devotes distinct chapters on personal stories of mental illness, thus validating the significance of cultural background and unique personal traits alongside objective symptoms.

Subject to a range of revisions in four preceding editions and a review process made public through a website www.DSM-5.org the current revision process was labelled as more open and democratic. In rectifying several limitations of the previous edition (DSM-IV), DSM-5 strived toward a more dynamic concept of culture. DSM-IV had de-emphasised the significance of social contexts and depicted "culture as residing largely within individuals" (Lopez and Guarnaccia 574). Most definitions also tend to portray culture as a static phenomenon and do not clarify how individuals negotiate various cultural spheres. In this context, the revisions in DSM-5 were lauded for its inclusivity and broadness. For instance, DSM-5 deeply elaborates how culture should be understood:

> Culture refers to systems of knowledge, concepts, rules, and practices that are learned and transmitted across generations. Culture includes language, religion and spirituality, family structures, life-cycle stages, ceremonial rituals, and customs, as well as moral and legal systems. Cultures are open, dynamic systems that undergo continuous change over time; in the contemporary world, most individuals and groups are exposed to multiple cultures, which they use to fashion their own identities and make sense of experience. These features of culture make it crucial not to overgeneralize cultural information or stereotype groups in terms of fixed cultural traits.
>
> (American Psychiatric Association, *Diagnostic* 749)

As such, the APA has commented that its fifth edition "incorporates a greater cultural sensitivity throughout the manual" (qtd. in Bredström 348). However, the manual tends to be read as a representative voice of authoritative musings on mental illness and is accepted globally as the rule book for diagnosing mental disorders. Despite these claims, there are prevailing criticisms against DSM-5 as a 'fiction' which medicalise human experience (Hicks). Gary Greenberg in his *The Book of Woe: The DSM and the Unmaking of Psychiatry* argues that "by imposing a pseudoscientific model on our 'hopelessly complex' inner world, it creates a 'charade' of non-existent disorders" (qtd. in Hicks). Moreover, the latest edition of the DSM which claims to be more inclusive of socio-cultural contexts and the distinctions across ethnic boundaries risks being relevant only for some patients. The latest edition still subscribes to static notions of culture by specifying certain symptoms as 'universal' and others as 'culturally specific expressions.' For instance, in case of panic attacks, 'uncontrollable crying and headaches' were listed as culturally specific while 'difficulty breathing' was listed as the primary/universal symptom (American Psychiatric Association, "Cultural Concepts").

From the above observations, it can be argued that the question of culture is yet not adequately addressed in DSM disorders or definitions. Essentialist, ethnocentric, and reductionist perspectives on illness experiences still permeate discourses surrounding mental health. As Pearce rightly argues, the use of scales and categories "lends the appearance of objectivity to a record of the patient's experience, but comes with the risk of abstraction from the patient experience in terms of narrative and context" (515). However, Foucault's genealogical perspectives on mental illness and institutions align with the voice of the vulnerable subjects in the clinical equation even in contemporary clinical settings. Foucault analyses how society conceived the defining attributes of the mentally ill throughout history in his seminal book *Madness and Civilization: A History of Insanity in the Age of Reason*. Focussing on the Renaissance to the twentieth century, Foucault observes that the figure of the *madman* had shifted from being an insider to an outsider from society. Consequently, the *insane* became an outcast that must be confined, studied, and treated as a medical object. As part of this historic evolution, asylums were established which were meant to *discipline* the subject kept under the supervision and authority of the doctor. Later, with the intervention of positivist concerns in medicine and psychiatry, these regiments of power operated in less visible forms. Even in the contemporary medical discourse, symptomatic and categorical prescriptions on mental illness naturalise the authority of medical voice over plural expressions of the illness experience. For instance, Foucault's view of madness as "a reification of a magical nature" (276) which implies the translation of a concept into an object correlates with objectives of modern psychiatry. As such, madness is not treated as an abstraction that can be used to make sense of reality, but as a biological reality that in reductive terms awaits clinical detection. The DSM-based diagnoses, in particular, ratify such reification as recent studies connote to diagnostic categories of the DSM are "nothing but conventional groupings of symptoms" (Vanheule). Umbrella terms used to designate a collection of symptoms, thus, get popularised as disease conditions that cause these symptoms, consequently affecting laymen and blinding professionals towards the subjective dimensions of mental illness.

An overview of diagnoses and treatment of the mentally ill reveals a range of practices and beliefs that centred on the autonomy of the healer and the vulnerability of the patient whose identity across centuries shifted from being an insider to an outcast lodged in isolated asylums. In the Middle Ages, the mentally ill were considered to have been possessed by evil spirits thus trapped in a supernatural phenomenon. Such perceptions led to bizarre treatment methods like trephining, a treatment procedure which included chipping a hole or trephine into the skull to create an opening that would release evil spirits and thus cure the person's psychopathology (Ellis et al. 176). In many cultures, mental illness is perceived as divine punishment imposed on a person who committed a sin against God and, therefore, as something an individual had imposed on himself. Consequently, the mentally ill were treated with religious rituals to drive out evil spirits which included exorcisms, incantations, and prayer. Also, the perception of mental illness as moral weakness resulted in patients being jailed as criminals and often put to death (Corrigan and Watson 37). The belief about mental illness was later altered by the Greek physician Hippocrates, who rejected the supernatural perspectives about mental illness and argued that psychological symptoms have natural causes, just like physical symptoms. Institutions like the Bethlem Hospital that isolated the 'insane' in the thirteenth century, to the Salpêtrière Hospital that was built in the seventeenth century, grew in number and sophistication. The close of the eighteenth century witnessed paradigm shifts regarding mental illness in parts of Europe. 'Mad-houses' where the 'violent' and 'dangerous' were accommodated changed to 'asylums' where the mentally ill could be treated and brought back as functional individuals in society ("History of Mental Illness").

Several studies have demonstrated how those with mental illness still suffer from social and perceived stigma (Bryne 1; Crisp et al. 6; Heginbotham 1052). Psychiatric labels that discriminate the mentally ill from the rest of the society cause social stigma, characterised by prejudicial attitudes and discriminating behaviour. On the other hand, when the sufferers of discrimination internalise the feelings of shame, it is referred to as perceived stigma or self-stigma leading to poorer treatment outcomes (Perlick et al. 1632). Etymologically, the word 'stigma' comes from the Greek word 'stigmata' which refers to "a mark of shame or discredit; a stain, or an identifying mark or characteristic" ("Stigma, noun"). In reference to mental illness, stigma is a multifaceted construct that involves attitudes, behaviours, and feelings. It is "a collection of negative attitudes, beliefs, thoughts, and behaviours that influences the individual, or the general public, to fear, reject, avoid, be prejudiced, and discriminate against people with mental disorders" (Gary 980). Moreover, stigma acts as a mediating process which legitimises and normalises discrimination and violence against people suffering from mental illness. Studies demonstrates that most people approached those with mental illness with caution and "fear of the mentally ill remains prevalent" (Rössler 1250). Such negative impressions often persist in people across cultures despite most of them being aware of the travails of mental illness through witnessing the illness condition in close familial and social circles. More recent studies (Pescosolido et al. 1736; Wang and Lai 192) reveal that a significant proportion of the public considered that people with mental illnesses such as depression or schizophrenia were unpredictable and dangerous, and they would be less likely to employ someone with a mental health problem.

As such, the mentally ill are labelled as deviants by society, as dysfunctional individuals in the framework of a society. Becker remarks, "[s]ocial groups create deviance by making the rules when infraction constitutes deviance and by applying their rules to particular people and labelling them as outsiders" (9). As the mentally ill inhabit an alternate reality, it is assumed that they are naturally bound to break the rules of a particular society. Ironically, the understanding of what constitutes 'abnormality' differs from one society to another; in other words, what is abnormal for one society or culture may be normal for another. However, Kleinman argues that mental health professionals themselves, family members, and sufferers are often the most effective and efficient transmitters of stigma due to factors such as poor conditions of care and social/financial burdens of care (603). Stigma in psychiatric institutions results in serious abuse of the mentally ill as evidenced in several studies: use of "unmodified electroconvulsive therapy"; violence, including sexual violence "against adults and children ... by staff or fellow patients" (Patel et al. 367). Furthermore, seclusion and isolation, as well as passivisation and inactivity of patients in psychiatric institutions, amplify the obstacles to patients' subsequent participation in the ordinary life and everyday social experience (Patel et al. 367).

## Mental Health Stigma and Medical Illustrations

The field of biomedicine is not immune to the popular beliefs about mental illness. According to Corrigan and Watson (2002) and Hugo (2001), most mental health professionals also subscribe to negative stereotypes about mental illness. Statistical surveys conducted as part of their study have revealed that medical professional groups were less optimistic about prognosis and long-term outcomes in this regard. People with mental illness are commonly viewed as 'weak, unproductive, and blameworthy' by many of the health professionals who treat them (Hinshaw 211). Such stigmatising experiences include

> feeling excluded from decisions, receiving subtle or overt threats of coercive treatment, being made to wait excessively long when seeking help, being given insufficient information about one's condition or treatment options, being treated in a paternalistic or demeaning manner, being told they would never get well, and being spoken to or about using stigmatizing language.
>
> (Knaak et al. 111)

The dehumanising approach of mental health professionals not only contributes to the stigma (Penn and Martin) but also results in worsening the condition of the ill (Sadow et al.). As patients and their families are often blamed for the mental health conditions that they suffer, Hinshaw argues that "stigmatization of the very people being served was built into the theoretical foundations of the mental health profession almost from the time of its formal establishment" (212).

Although inhuman treatment practices in asylums could be linked to the cultural factors that shaped physicians' prejudice towards the mentally ill as impassive exiles from a 'normal,' functional society, the typology of illustrated histories of medicine legitimised such attitudes. Sander Gilman in his seminal investigation of the illustrated histories of mental illness traces several examples that reflected the cultural history of madness and legitimised its claims in academic psychiatry. Gilman in *Seeing the Insane* (1982) and *Picturing Health and Illness: Images of Identity and Difference* (1995) critically examines visual representations of the mentally ill across centuries as "cultural fantasies of health, disease, and the body" (*Picturing* 18). Gilman unveils the selection and editing involved in choosing visual representations of the mentally ill and claims that the use of pictures in medical texts cannot be deemed as naïve but highly manipulative. The overarching claim of these representations, Gilman argues, is that there is no internal reality to be examined, only the external world internalised and represented in art (*Picturing* 19). Irrespective of the medium—illustrations or photographs—these visual representations emphasised the need for the psychiatrists to *see* the patient and his/her signs and symptoms as the key to diagnosis. Intriguingly, such medical iconography was not distinct from the presumptions of madness in the general iconography of Western representational art (*Seeing* 24). As such, the field of psychiatry was obsessed with creating a visual epistemology from which the subjectivity of the patient was completely absent. As Gilman observes:

'Picturing' is moved from being an individual act in a historical context, to that of the collective self-labelled as 'scientists' without much consideration to the mechanisms present. ... It is, as Peter Novick argued, decades ago, the creation of an academic notion of objectivity out of the subjectivity of the historical agent.

("Representing")

As such, these visual representations influence medical perceptions of the mentally ill binding the general misconceptions and anxieties about madness. Most representations followed the beauty/ugly binary based on the patient's physiognomic features. By the close of the eighteenth century, the association of madness with specific physiognomy had become commonplace in European thought. Although Phillippe Pinel is highly regarded for introducing humane treatment and reform in French asylums, he is also instrumental in altering perspectives on psychopathology. In his *Treatise on Insanity* (1801), Pinel included two images comparing the shape of the skull of two patients. The analysis further developed to include comparisons with the ideal proportions of Greek sculpture thus measuring the physiognomy of the mentally ill on the plane of aesthetic perceptions (Gilman, *Seeing* 73).

Such perceptions even led various psychiatrists to propose comparisons with the physiognomy of animals to perceive the mental status of their patients and to distinguish them from the ideal structure of a normal person. For instance, August Krauss' table of animal analogues demonstrates how madness was perceived in terms of patient's physiognomic features (*Picturing* 37). Hidden implications of such parallels drawn between physiognomic ugliness and mental impairment connote to the construction of categories of beauty/health and ugliness/illness (*Picturing* 38). In fact, these essential categories may cater to the aesthetics of a particular group or class as well as specific individual aesthetics of the time. Here, Krauss' question of physiognomy and the features of the various breeds of horse could be read as encoded in the cultural ethos of science in the nineteenth century. In this context, Gilman rightly comments on the necessity to keenly observe the nuanced braiding of the public and private reveries of mental illness thus:

The role of the study of medical (in the broadest sense) representations, or perhaps better, images of health and illness and their attendant social and cultural settings needs to be addressed ... The function of representations (and those trained to study and analyze them) in the history of medicine is to knit the function of

public and private representations with the continuities and dis-
continuities in attitudes and beliefs both within and beyond the
health sciences.

("Representing")

These prejudiced manifestations of the mentally ill not only affected
the physician's attitude towards the mentally ill, but also precipitated
negative metaphors in the cultural discourse on mental illness. In this
context, online initiatives by groups such as the Cochrane Common
Mental Disorders Group (CCMD) (based at the University of York,
UK) seek to reconfigure prevalent stereotypes used in medical blog
posts and clinical resources. Jessica Hendon, the Managing Editor of
CCMD, in her recent article, "Picturing Mental Health: What Sort of
Images Are the Right Ones?", reflects on the middle ground of representing mental illness. Instead of exaggerating the benefits or harms of
the treatment or promoting positive images of mental health that focus
on prevention and recovery, Hendon bats for 'lived experiences' and
how it should inform representations of mental illnesses over corporate or clichéd versions of mental conditions.

## Conjuring Stereotypes through Media Representations

As in medical discourse, a tendency to visualise mental illness in stock
patterns also exists within art and popular culture. A careful analysis
of the history of visual representations of the mentally ill reveals a
set of repeated stereotyped ideas/images from the sixteenth century
to contemporary popular culture. Cumulatively, these representations
of the mentally ill reflect the dominant attitudes and behaviours towards them, that is, a constant fear of the Other. Further, they also
reinforce the presumed boundaries between normal and abnormal.
The stereotypical cultural representation of the diseased body and its
psychological manifestation as a dangerous Other is reflected in illness
discourses across time.

In making a clear distinction between the ill and the healthy, several representations in art also characterise the mentally ill as animals
devoid of human qualities. As Foucault remarks, "madness had become a thing to look at: no longer a monster inside oneself, but an
animal with strange mechanisms, a bestiality from which man had
long since been suppressed" (66). Foucault's observation unveils the
predominant cultural logic of considering the 'mad' as a beast which
must be confined and controlled. One of the earliest examples of meta-
phorising madness as animalistic is reflected in Charles Bell's *Madman*

(1806). The image reflects the larger cultural anxiety of not being able to identify a person with mental illness and feeds the desire to alienate them from the 'normal' society. The 'madman's' glance directed away from the readers characterised by indignant gestures suggests unpredictability and impending danger. Like an untamed animal, the 'madman' with dishevelled hair is chained and left naked. Interestingly, the image reciprocates the predominant Middle Age fantasies about madness. Such persistent notions about the mentally ill reflect the cultural preoccupations of controlling and taming the undesirable Other in conspicuous ways despite centuries of evolved scientific and cultural perceptions about mental illness.

Sensationalisation and stigmatisation of mental illness are also evident in popular media representations. Perpetuating stereotypes and capitalising on the increased anxiety, several negative and inaccurate portrayals of mental illness influence the public perception of mental illness. Most movies deploy illness as a trope of violence and crime. Horror movies often include scary and dangerous slashers who suffer from psychosis. Alfred Hitchcock's *Psycho* (1960), for instance, features Anthony Perkins as Norman Bates who kills a female motel guest. The scene of the murder captures the gruesome details of the slashing and the helplessness of the female victim, Marion, enacted by Janet Leigh. Norman Bates is not identified as a mental patient until the end of the film when a psychiatrist explains the origins of his bizarre behaviour.

Since *Psycho*, slasher movies that peaked in popularity in the late 1970s and continued through the 1980s and beyond improvise the same theme. The elements of violence and fear are exaggerated with dramatic special effects in these movies. Otto F. Wahl in *Media Madness: Public Images of Mental Illness* observes that mentally ill characters in movies and different television shows were more likely to be villains who were undeniably violent. The adjectives that best describe the mentally ill in these representations were "active," "confused," "aggressive," "dangerous," and "unpredictable" (Wahl 66).

Several studies by Wahl et al. and Wilson et al., have also shown that portrayals of the mentally ill are mostly negative and thus perpetuate stereotypes about mental illness. Even in technical details such as framing and point of view, these filmic representations convey that the mentally ill are different from other characters. Moreover, pejorative terms such as 'crazy,' 'psycho,' 'deranged,' and 'loony' are often used by other characters in reference to the mentally ill (Wahl et al. 554; Wilson et al. 441). Apart from *Psycho*, many films such as Miloš Forman's *One Flew Over the Cuckoo's Nest* (1975) and Tony

Bill's *Crazy People* (1990) exploit such terms to intrigue and entertain the viewer. The characters themselves are often portrayed with distinctive and unattractive features like rotting teeth or unruly hair (Wilson et al. 442). In exploring television images of madness, Simon Cross studies "Whose Mind Is It Anyway" a British television show, which aims to present the implications of releasing mental patients from asylums. Each shot fully exploits the standard icons of dangerous insanity in the patient's crooked facial expressions and dishevelled appearances. The presenter explains to viewers that a "mentally disturbed man has been seen brandishing a knife at a local restaurant" (141). The next shot presents a police car with the siren sounding, moving at speed to catch the dangerously insane. Such negative images of violence and control permeate most filmic representations of the mentally ill. Although certain movies like *A Beautiful Mind* (2001) and *They Look Like People* (2015) provide sympathetic and honest portrayals of mental illness, recent films such as *Bug* (2006), *Split* (2016), and *Birdbox* (2018) also draw icons from the violent stereotype of madness. Jane Pirkis and others in "On-Screen Portrayals of Mental Illness: Extent, Nature, and Impacts" categorise such stereotypes from filmic representations thus: the homicidal maniac, the rebellious free spirit, the female patient as a seductress, the narcissistic parasite, and the zoo specimen (528–529). As such, these portrayals reduce the mentally ill to essentially negative categories. In a different vein, few filmic representations also perpetuate unscientific and unrealistic notions about mental illness and coping strategies. *Silver Linings Playbook* (2012), for instance, presents unrealistic ways of managing bipolar disorder. Although the first half of the movie bluntly portrays the dysfunction of the characters and the travails of bipolar disorder on the family, it over-emphasises an easy recovery when the two main characters engage in a romantic relationship. *The Visit* (2015) also inaccurately portrays those with schizophrenia as struggling with murderous tendencies. The mentally ill characters in the movie are represented as inherently dangerous with odd behaviours, hallucinations, and paranoia.

Comics, "the only proximate medium of film" (Chute, *Graphic Women* 221) is also not excluded from such negative/distorted images of mental illness. Alan Moore and Dave Gibbon's *Watchmen,* for instance, presents characters like Rorschach, the Incredible Hulk, and David "Legion" Haller as victims of trauma and is often marginalised and socially excluded. Within such an environment, their mental health problems unsurprisingly worsen.

Rorschach is dismissed as paranoid and crazy by his fellow costumed adventurers, leading him to spiral downward until he believes violent murder to be the only viable option in his war on crime. The Hulk is ostracized for being a monster and becomes even more dangerous the more isolated he gets.

(Langley)

Similarly, *Batman* series also reinforces the violent stereotype of insanity in characters like Two-Face (split personality disorder) and The Joker (Psychopath) who set the standard for a typical villain in most comic books that followed. The *New York Times* published an article by psychiatrists H. Eric Bender et al. in 2011 that challenged the distorted representations of the mentally ill in DC comics:

[W]hen contemporary psychiatric terms or disorders have been used in stories, they have been misapplied to explain villainy. As Grant Morrison, a well-known comic author, wrote recently, "The rest of Batman's rogues' gallery personified various psychiatric disorders to great effect: Two-Face was [represented as suffering from] schizophrenia." But Two-Face's central quality, a split personality, isn't characteristic of schizophrenia. Similarly, the Joker is often called "psychotic," despite a lack of hallucinations or other symptoms of a psychotic disorder. True, some say, "these are just comic books." But such inaccuracies perpetuate harmful stereotypes.

Sensationalised media reports of real events also influence the public perception about the mentally ill. Research indicates that most news reports represent the mentally ill as violent and criminal than benign or sympathetic (Wahl 67). Along with the prevalent notion of the mentally ill as fundamentally flawed and evil rather than as an ill person, news reports frequently suggest that those with mental illness cannot be cured completely despite treatment. Catering to the common plot pattern of the mentally ill who are bent on terrorising the innocent, these reports demonstrate the ineffectiveness of treatment for the mentally ill. For instance, newspaper reports like the one published in *the New York Post* on 9 May 1982, confirm that former patients will be prone to violence even after treatment. The catchy headline "Freed Mental Patient Kills Mom" in bold capital letters provokes the readers to assume that those once labelled as mentally ill must be approached with caution. As such, the patients continue to experience the stigma of exclusion and violence throughout their lives even after being medically cured.

Reports on the mentally ill as the dangerous Other and the deliberate use of phrases like 'crazy' in describing the mentally ill further reinforce the negative stereotypes and metaphors that dehumanise the mentally ill. In other words, such reiterated usages diminish the 'credibility, trustworthiness, and value' of the person suffering from mental illness (Wahl et al. 559). Biased and sensationalised reports as such mislead the public by portraying the mentally ill as aggressive, dangerous, and unpredictable. A recent study by Marian Chen and Stephen Lawrie reveals that "only 5% of the homicides carried out in the general population between 2001 and 2011 were by those with an abnormal mental state" (309). Also, it is found that those with mental disorder are more inclined to self-harm than harm others. Despite these facts, news media perpetuates sensationalist notions about mental illness that dehumanise patients to the extent that they are defined by these presumed symptoms of their illness.

When media representations of schizophrenia present false perceptions, even medical definitions about mental illness may not serve the full purpose of redeeming the validity of one's lived experience of illness. W. J. T. Mitchell in a lecture titled "What Do Pictures Want" argues that madness, as represented in popular media, is not necessarily at the periphery of human experience. Departing from the medical symptomatic definitions of schizophrenia, Mitchell presents an alternate yet valid perspective about the illness which is unavailable in popular representations of schizophrenia:

> schizophrenia can be understood as an intensified form of normal mental activity of the work of reason, memory, and imagination spinning out of control; the perfectly ordinary process of inner vision and audition exaggerated so that fantasy take on a tactile and visceral reality.

His deliberate choice of the words 'normal,' 'ordinary,' and 'reality' reflects an attempt to free madness from its confinement in the discourse of medicine and popular culture as an abnormal and exotic abstraction.

Reinforced by different media representations, dehumanised metaphors of violence and idiocy permeate into everyday language and slang words which connote to mental illness. As advertisements aim to attract the viewers' attention, they often deploy slang terms and offensive images of mental illness. Especially, advertisements for peanuts engage in a wordplay on the double meaning of 'nuts.' For instance, a particular peanut product was packed as a gift bag in a straightjacket labelled 'Certifiably Nuts.' The package was branded with a 'patient history' stating that the owner's family had been 'nuts for generations.' Although tags such as these imply the quality of the product as time-tested, they subtly convey unscientific notions about hereditary links to mental illness (Davidson). Additionally, pulling a string attached to the peanut package would release a hysterical laughter, a charac-teristic drawn from stereotyped representations of the mentally ill as idiotic. The product and the advertisement tags serve as metaphors of mental illness which construe and perpetuate negative and stereo-typed perceptions about those suffering from mental illness.

Consistency in the negative representations of mental illness in ad-vertisements reinforces the stereotyped perspectives on mental illness. Most visual representations of the mentally ill in advertisements em-phasise distinctive physical features. Caricatured wild eyes and un-kempt hair, in particular, are the defining traits of the mentally ill in these portrayals. Such distinctions underscore the politics involved in the selection of images despite the fact that the reality of mental illness is varied and more human.

Although metaphors are often inconspicuously deployed in rep-resentations of illness, Elaine Scarry observes that metaphors do not merely function as rhetorical devices but as tools imbued with ideol-ogies that configure popular perceptions about illness. Scarry in *The Body in Pain* discusses how the experience of pain is articulated in language exclusively through metaphors of weaponry and damage (15). Similarly, Susan Sontag in *Illness as Metaphor* traces metaphors that conceptualise disease as an "evil, invincible predator" (7). Trac-ing several figurative uses of diseases as a metaphor for monstrosity and destructiveness in nineteenth-century literature, Sontag attempts to reveal its origin in social prejudices and stereotypes. Sontag clari-fies how military metaphors "contribute to the stigmatizing of certain illnesses and by extension, of those who are ill" (97).

In the context of mental illness, popular media like movies and ad-vertisements configure several metaphors as identified by Scarry and Sontag. Advertisements on mental health, for instance, often follow a tragedy narrative with sad faces in dim background and lighting which stereotype mental illnesses like depression as a uniform experi-ence. Worse still are pharmaceutical advertisements where metaphors of sadness and gloom prevail until the patient is medicated with a particular drug. These advertisements portray medication as a sole method of dealing with mental illnesses. Accordingly, these advertise-ments reconfigure the background setting with metaphors of hope and happiness. For instance, S. E. Smith refers to early advertisements on

Prozac®, a drug used for treating depression, which features characters who engage in heavy-handed metaphors like opening the blinds to 'let the sunshine in.' In averting the mental health condition, Smith observes, "[p]atients should just take a pill ... according to the narrative in pharmaceutical advertising, when the truth can be more complicated." Such portrayals shadow the significance of mental support that friends and family provide the mentally ill by emphasising medication which impacts patients differently and is not the only path to recovery.

Against such stereotyped representations of mental illness, Sue Estroff argues that mental illness cannot be reduced to an object; it is not "something that someone *has* and that is external to whomever is experiencing it" (qtd. in Vanthuyne 413). On the contrary, the experience of mental illness is "socially situated, individualized version of a body of cultural knowledge" (Vanthuyne 413). However, the different cultural idioms and stereotypes that are hierarchically positioned within a network of power relationships constitute deleterious metaphors of mental illness which appropriate subjective experiences to popular expectations. A close analysis of the visual representations of mental illness across popular media reveals the visual attributes and nuances that construct metaphoric meanings that have deleterious impact on those suffering from the illness. Similarly, metaphors of mental illness that circulate in medical discourse through psychiatric idioms prevent the mentally ill and their community from exploring the diverse socio-political perspectives of living with mental illness. In this context, Aristotle's contention proves significant: "Metaphors, like epithets, must be fitting, which means they must fairly correspond to the thing signified: failing this, their inappropriateness will be conspicuous" (2240).

## Conclusion

Popular and non-popular representations of mental illness (such as paintings, movies, news reports, advertisements, cartoons, and medical discourse) wield a rhetorical power, in that they influence perceptions about the illness and those who suffer from it. Patient's internal reality is constructed and reconstructed through the representations which very often align with the market demands, cultural expectations, and extant stereotypes. Negative and inaccurate representations of mental illness in art, medicine, and popular media thus serve as a means of controlling the boundaries of normality, acceptability, and inclusivity. The prejudices perpetuated towards the mentally ill and the stigma that it engenders influence the societal attitudes towards those suffering from mental illness. Therefore, in the absence of personal accounts of illness or accurate representations of patients' subjective reality, the mentally ill would be subject to systematic exclusion from civic and social life.

Furthermore, the representations of the mentally ill as violent and unpredictable in popular media have adverse effects on diverse domains of the patient's life. Approached with caution and distrust, these individuals would continue to live with shame and guilt despite being cured of illness. As such, the label of mental illness, the exaggerated and grossly distorted representations of it, and the self-stigma and public stigma induced by it subtly influence their intra-subjective and inter-subjective realities.

## Acknowledgement

This chapter is derived in part from an article published in *Media Watch*. See Ventakesan, Sathyaraj, and Sweetha Saji. "Conjuring the 'Insane': Representations of Mental Illness in Medical and Popular Discourses." *Media Watch*, vol. 10, no. 3, 2019, pp. 522–538. Available at https://www.mediawatchjournal.in/conjuring-the-insane-representations-of-mental-illness-in-medical-and-popular-discourses/.

## Reference List

American Psychiatric Association. "Cultural Concepts in DSM-5." *American Psychiatric Association*, 2013. PDF File.
———. *Diagnostic and Statistical Manual of Mental Disorders: DSM-5*. American Psychiatric Association, 2013.
Andreasen, Nancy C. "DSM and the Death of Phenomenology in America: An Example of Unintended Consequences." *Schizophrenia Bulletin*, vol. 33, no. 1, 2007, pp. 108–112.
Aristotle. "Rhetoric." *The Complete Works of Aristotle: The Revised Oxford Translation*, edited by Jonathan Barnes, Princeton UP, 1984, pp. 2152–2269.
Baldonado, Ann Marie. "Representation." Fall 1996. *Postcolonial Studies at Emory Pages*, October 2017, https://scholarblogs.emory.edu/postcolonialstudies/2014/06/21/representation/.
Becker, Howard S. *Outsiders: Studies in the Sociology of Deviance*. The Free P, 1963.
Bender, H. Eric, et al. "Putting the Caped Crusader on the Couch." *The New York Times*, 20 September 2011, https://www.nytimes.com/2011/09/21/opinion/putting-the-caped-crusader-on-the-couch.html.
Bredström, Anna. "Culture and Context in Mental Health Diagnosing: Scrutinizing the DSM-5 Revision." *Journal of Medical Humanities*, vol. 40, 2019, pp. 347–363.

Bryne, Peter. "Stigma of Mental Illness: Changing Minds, Changing Behaviour." *The British Journal of Psychiatry*, vol. 174, no. 1, 1999, pp. 1–2.

Chen, Marian, and Stephen Lawrie. "Newspaper Depictions of Mental and Physical Health." *BJPsych Bulletin*, vol. 41, no. 6, 2017, pp. 308–313.

Chute, Hillary. *Graphic Women: Life Narrative and Contemporary Comics.* Columbia UP, 2010.

Corrigan, Patrick W., and Amy C. Watson. "The Paradox of Self-Stigma and Mental Illness." *Clinical Psychology: Science and Practice*, vol. 9, no. 1, 2002, pp. 35–53.

Crisp, Arthur H. et al. "Stigmatisation of People with Mental Illness." *The British Journal of Psychiatry: The Journal of Mental Science.* vol. 177, 2000, pp. 4–7.

Cross, Simon. *Mediating Madness: Mental Distress and Cultural Representation.* Palgrave Macmillan, 2010.

Davidson, Ashley. "Is Mental Illness Hereditary?" *HuffPost*, 30 May 2018, https://www.huffpost.com/entry/mental-illness-hereditary_n_5afb1035e 4b0200bcab93ffc.

Edgar, Andrew, and Peter Sedgwick. *Key Concepts in Cultural Theory.* Routledge, 2005.

Ellis, Albert, et al. *Personality Theories: Critical Perspectives.* Sage, 2009.

Foucault, Michel. *Madness and Civilization: A History of Insanity in the Age of Reason*, translated by Richard Howard. Random House, 2005.

Gary, Faye A. "Stigma: Barrier to Mental Health Care among Ethnic Minorities." *Issues in Mental Health Nursing*, vol. 26, no. 10, 2005, pp. 979–999.

Gilman, Sander L. *Picturing Health and Illness: Images of Identity and Difference.* Johns Hopkins UP, 1995.

———. "Representing Health and Illness: Thoughts for the 21st century." *Medical History*, vol. 55, no. 3, 2011, https://www.ncbi.nlm.nih.gov/pmc/articles/PMC3143852/.

———. *Seeing the Insane.* 1982. Echo Point, 2014.

Hall, Stuart. *Representations: Cultural Representations and Signifying Practices.* Sage, 1997.

Heginbotham, Chris. "UK Mental Health Policy Can Alter the Stigma of Mental Illness." *The Lancet*, vol. 352, no. 9133, 1998, pp. 1052–1053.

Hendon. Jessica. "Picturing Mental Health: What Sort of Images Are the Right Ones?" *Evidently Cochrane*, 7 February 2020, https://www.evidently-cochrane.net/picturing-mental-health/.

Hicks, Cherrill. "Dozens of Mental Disorders Don't Exist." *The Telegraph*, 6 October 2013, https://www.telegraph.co.uk/news/health/10359105/Dozens-of-mental-disorders-dont-exist.html.

Hinshaw, Stephen P. *The Mark of Shame: Stigma of Mental Illness and an Agenda for Change.* Oxford UP, 2007.

"History of Mental Illness: An Overview." PDF File, https://shodhganga.inflibnet.ac.in/bitstream/10603/39127/7/07_chapter%202.pdf.

Horgan, John. "Psychiatry in Crisis! Mental Health Director Rejects Psychiatric "Bible" and Replaces with Nothing." *Scientific American*, 4 May 2013, https://

blogs.scientificamerican.com/cross-check/psychiatry-in-crisis-mental-healthdirector-rejects-psychiatric-bible-and-replaces-with-nothing/?-redirect=1.

Hugo, Malcolm. "Mental Health Professionals' Attitudes towards People Who Have Experienced a Mental Health Disorder." *Journal of Psychiatric and Mental Health Nursing*, vol. 8, no. 5, 2001, pp. 419–425.

Johnstone, Megan-Jane. "Stigma, Social Justice, and the Rights of the Mentally Ill: Challenging the Status Quo." *Australian and New Zealand Journal of Mental Health Nursing*, vol. 10, 2001, pp. 200–209.

Kleinman, Arthur. "Global Mental Health: A Failure of Humanity." *The Lancet*, vol. 374, no. 9690, 2009, pp. 603–604.

Knaak, Stephanie, et al. "Mental Illness-Related Stigma in Healthcare: Barriers to Access and Care and Evidence-Based Solutions." *Healthcare Management Forum*, vol. 30, no. 2, 2017, pp. 111–116.

Langley, Adam. "Superpowers, Mental Health, and the Problems of Representation." *Syfy Wire*, 9 April 2018, https://www.syfy.com/syfywire/superpowers-mental-health-and-the-problems-of-representation.

Lewis, Bradley. *Moving beyond Prozac, DSM, and the New Psychiatry: The Birth of Postpsychiatry*. The U of Michigan P, 2006.

Lopez, Steven R., and Peter J. J. Guarnaccia. "Cultural Psychopathology: Uncovering the Social World of Mental Illness." *Annual Review of Psychology*, vol. 51, no. 1, 2000, pp. 571–599.

Mitchell, W. J. T. *Picture Theory*. The U of Chicago P, 1994.

Myers, Bob Eberly. *"Drapetomania": Rebellion, Defiance and Free Black Insanity in the Antebellum United States*. U of California, 2014.

Patel, Vikarm, et al. "Protecting the Human Rights of People with Mental Illnesses: A Call to Action for Global Mental Health." *Mental Health and Human Rights: Vision, Praxis, and Courage*, edited by Michael Dudley, Derrick Silove & Fran Gale, Oxford UP, 2012, pp. 362–375.

Pearce, Steve. "DSM-5 and the Rise of the Diagnostic Checklist." *Journal of Medical Ethics*, vol. 40, no. 8, 2014, pp. 515–516.

Penn, David L., and James Martin. "The Stigma of Severe Mental Illness: Some Potential Solutions for a Recalcitrant Problem." *Psychiatric Quarterly*, vol. 69, no. 3, 1998, pp. 235–247.

Perlick, Deborah A., et al. "Stigma as a Barrier to Recovery: Adverse Effects of Perceives Stigma on Social Adaptation of Persons Diagnosed with Bipolar Affective Disorder." *Psychiatric Services*, vol. 52, no. 12, 2001, pp. 1627–1632.

Pescosolido, Bernice A., et al. "Evolving Public Views on the Likelihood of Violence from People with Mental Illness: Stigma and Its Consequences." *Health Affairs*, vol. 38, no. 10, 2019, pp. 1735–1743.

Pirkis, Jane, et al. "On-Screen Portrayals of Mental Illness: Extent, Nature, and Impacts." *Journal of Health Communication: International Perspectives*, vol. 11, no. 5, 2006, pp. 523–541.

Quayson, Ato. *Aesthetic Nervousness: Disability and the Crisis of Representation*. Columbia UP, 2007.

Rössler, Wulf. "The Stigma of Mental Disorders: A Millennia-Long History of Social Exclusion and Prejudices." *EMBO Reports*, vol. 17, no. 9, 2016, pp. 1250–1253.

Roth, Nancy L., and Katy Hogan. *Gendered Epidemic: Representations of Women in the Age of AIDS*. Routledge, 1998.

Sadow, Dolly, et al. "Is the Education of Health Professionals Encouraging Stigma towards Mentally Ill?" *Journal of Mental Health*, vol. 11, no. 6, 2002, pp. 657–665.

Said, Edward. "Orientalism." *The Edward Said Reader*, edited by Moustafa Bayoumi, and Andrew Rubin, Vintage, 2000, pp. 63–113.

Scarry, Elaine. *The Body in Pain: The Making and Unmaking of the World*. Oxford UP, 1985.

Shohat, Ella. "The Struggle over Representation: Casting, Coalitions, and the Politics of Identification." *Late Imperial Culture*, edited by Roman de la Campa, E. Ann Kaplan and Michael Sprinkler, Verso, 1995, pp. 166–178.

Smith, S. E. "We're All Mad Here: Pharmaceutical Advertising and Messaging about Mental Illness." *BitchMedia*, 29 August 2011, https://www.bitchmedia.org/post/were-all-mad-here-pharmaceutical-advertising-and-messaging-about-mental-illness.

Sontag, Susan. *Illness as Metaphor: AIDS and Its Metaphors*. Penguin, 1991.

"Stigma, noun." *Merriam-Webster Dictionary*, https://www.merriam-webster.com/dictionary/stigma.

Treichler, Paula A. *How to Have Theory in an Epidemic: Cultural Chronicles of AIDS*. Duke UP, 2006.

Vanheule, Stijn. "What Can We Learn from Michel Foucault?" *Global Summit on Diagnostic Alternatives*, 30 April 2014, http://dxsummit.org/archives/2055.

Vanthuyne, Karine. "Searching for the Words to Say It: The Importance of Cultural Idioms in the Articulation of the Experience of Mental Illness." *Ethos,* vol. 31, no. 3, 2003, pp. 412–433.

Wahl, Otto F. *Media Madness: Public Images of Mental Illness*. 1995. Rutgers UP, 2003.

Wahl, Otto F., et al. "Mental Illness Depiction in Children's Films." *Journal of Community Psychology*, vol. 31, no. 6, 2003, pp. 553–560.

Wang, Jainli, and Daniel W. L. Lai. "The Relationship between Mental Health Literacy, Personal Contacts, and Personal Stigma against Depression." *Journal of Affective Disorders*, vol. 110, no. 1–2, 2008, pp. 191–196.

"What do Pictures Want? Lecture by William J. Thomas Mitchell." *YouTube*, uploaded by Muzeum, 4 November 2012, https://www.youtube.com/watch?v=VHe9pWSUIjg.

Wilson, C., et al. "How Mental Illness Is Portrayed in Children's Television." *The British Journal of Psychiatry: The Journal of Mental Science*, vol. 176, no. 5, 2000, pp. 440–443.

# 4 Nobody Memoirs as Counter-Discourse

## Bipolar Disorder and Its Metaphors

## Introduction

Medical and popular discourses, as discussed in the previous chapter ("Mental Illness and the Politics of Representation"), often perpetuate stereotypes of the mentally ill that essentialise them as imbecile and violent, which in turn trivialises their voices and perspectives (Boysen et al. 353; O'Hern 68). Because of this, stereotyped representations of mental illness mediated through films, fiction, or pedagogical texts often follow a pattern of exclusion (Felman 13). Personal narratives of mental illness, on the contrary, restore the language of mental illness as experienced by the mentally ill and therefore challenge and subvert the dominant representations. In this context, graphic memoirs of mental illness are a cultural resource in redeeming the identity and truths of those suffering from mental illness. The genre takes effect rhetorically through stylistic techniques and metaphors that critique normative conceptualisations of the behavioural patterns of the mentally ill. Taking these cues, this chapter explores the diverse ways in which graphic memoirs on mental illness construct a counter-discourse by challenging and subverting the stereotypical representations of mental illness. Specifically, through a close-reading of Ellen Forney's *Marbles: Mania, Depression, Michelangelo, and Me* (2012) (hereafter *Marbles*) and of Rachel Lindsay's *Rx: A Graphic Memoir* (2018) (hereafter *Rx*), which deftly describe the subjective realities of bipolar disorder, this chapter investigates the role and function of metaphors (visual/verbo-visual) as a tool of counter-diagnosis.[1] This chapter also seeks to address the following questions: (a) how does the author's own visual narrative renegotiate and renew cultural and medical perceptions of these bodies/minds which have been distorted by popular media representations and oiomedical prescriptions of mental disorders? (b) what form of agency is entailed in wielding control

DOI: 10.4324/9781003214229-5

over the representation of self-image and deconstruction of the sanity/ insanity binary?

Building on the extant notions of mental illness, cultural representations of bipolar disorder are replete with negative perceptions and stereotypes surrounding the illness. For instance, *Mr. Jones*, which appeared in 1993, directed by Mike Figgis, portrays a love relationship between a lady psychiatrist and her bipolar patient. Although the movie has been acclaimed for its insights on euphoria, mania, and depression, its marketing tagline, "everything that makes him dangerous makes her love him more," reproduces the metaphoric association of the mentally ill as violent and dangerous. Similarly, several short films uploaded on social media platforms like *YouTube* that claim to represent bipolar disorder have been critiqued by viewers marking their disapproval through their comments. Even in technical details, such as framing and point of view, these representations convey that the mentally ill are different from other characters. For instance, a short film titled "Bipolar" by Janis Jurgelis and Joshua Behrens, which was uploaded to *YouTube* on 17 October 2013, utilises skewed camera angles and predominantly dim lighting techniques, which in turn accelerates the mystery surrounding bipolar disorder. The short film, towards the end, draws inaccurate parallels between split personality and bipolar disorder as the protagonist appears both as the patient and as the doctor. Although it gained over 800,000 views, several viewers have commented that it does not portray the reality of bipolar disorder and that it is poorly researched.[2] In his analysis of stereotypes of bipolar disorder in television shows from the twenty-first century, Declan O'Hern argues that instances of violence and criminal behaviour were presented frequently (71). Additionally, television shows such as *Degrassi*, *Homeland*, *Shameless*, and *Empire* represented bipolar patients as violent while in reality only 11%–16% of bipolar patients experience violent episodes (Vann).

Comics also perpetuate negative/distorted images of bipolar disorder. Both DC and Marvel comics limn bipolar characters either as creative and intelligent (for example, Dr William Magnus in DC's *Metal Men*) or as villainous (for example, Aquarius in DC's *Justice League of America*) and tag-along tricksters (for example, James Jesse in DC's "Flash and Substance"). James Jesse, for instance, is not even portrayed as a serious villain because he has bipolar disorder and is often disregarded by his team ("11 superheroes"). Such trivialisation of bipolar characters in mainstream comics not only reinforces the violent stereotype of insanity and instigates discrimination against bipolar patients, but also perpetuates pseudo notions about bipolar condition.

Such stereotypical representations, which force viewers to assume agitation and aggression as common symptoms of bipolar disorder, are also prevalent cross-culturally. The 2006 Malayalam movie *Vadakkunnathan,* directed by Shajoon Kariyal, revolves around the life of a college professor who suffers from bipolar disorder.[3] Most of the protagonist's psychic turmoil in the movie is filmed either during the night or in dimly lit corridors. As observed by Koravangattu Menon and Gopinath Ranjith, the movie does not show any characteristic symptoms of mania or depression although the protagonist claims to be bipolar (220). Catering to the stereotyped portrayals of mental illness, the character is also shown as having hallucinations, which is a clinically inaccurate representation of bipolar disorder. Ratnakaran et al. have shown that several other Malayalam movies on bipolar disorder, like the 2013 films *Left Right Left* and *Silence* and the 2018 film *Hey Jude,* also fail to represent the pervasive mood shifts characteristic of the disorder.

In this context, personal narratives of bipolar disorder critically reconfigure such prejudiced misconceptions particularly through metaphors that encapsulate authors' unique experiences. Besides challenging the popular notions of vulnerability and monstrosity, subjective accounts of mental conditions develop a parallel discourse from marginal perspectives that very often challenge, subvert, ironically mimic, or creatively play with extant stereotypes. *Marbles* and *Rx* are such cultural texts that "resist subjugation and voice positions of non-normalcy" (Longhurst 38).

## Personal Stories, Memoirs, and Counter-Discourse

As a variant form of life writing, memoir recalls specific events from one's or another's life. In Thomas Couser's terms, memoirs reflect the nature of a life narrative which develops through social networks and interpersonal relationships (*Memoir* 20). Although other forms of life writing such as autobiographies claim to narrate entire events from a person's life to death, as Couser argues, "much self-life writing focuses only on a discrete part of life" (23). In the context of narratives about illness experience or disability, authors inevitably deal with a single-dimension of life, and hence, their narratives are more properly called memoir than autobiography.

Established since the Enlightenment, autobiographies focussed on one specific individual, the "sovereign self" (Smith and Watson 3). As such, writers who are qualified to be autobiographers comprise "a set of 'exemplary' literary, political, and military men; they have been seen (and this view persists) as singular figures capable of summing up an era in a name: Augustine, Rousseau, Franklin, Henry Adams" (Gilmore 11). This definition of the autobiographical subject elevated the status of the genre as a part of high culture. By the turn of the twentieth century, the marginalised were engaging in different forms of life writing although they were not accepted as part of the autobiography tradition. However, the field of autobiography began to expand since then to encompass life narratives transcending the boundaries of race, gender, and popularity. In recent years, critics of the genre have shifted their focus from the subject of autobiographies to questions of identity, power, and truth that are challenged and reconfigured through a range of self-representations of lived experiences. Accordingly, John Wiltshire argues that autobiographies about illness experiences are not simply aimed at representing an ideal self but are a result of a predicament which is thrust upon the author, which she/he explores in the narrative alongside a community of sufferers:

> Authors of pathographic narratives are different from ordinary biographers in one important sense: they are, as it were, reluctant. Their subject does not represent some ego-ideal, some alternative or companion selfhood in following whose footsteps one might (however obscurely, however indirectly) be exploring one's own choices or enhancing the sense of one's own possibilities. The subject of the pathographer's biography is not chosen, but appears to be devolved upon him or her by necessity.
>
> (414)

In a similar vein, arguing against reducing the complexities of mental illness into few externally visible stock features, Sue Estroff, one of the first ethnographers of mental health patients, proposes that the illness is not external to the patient but is "something that someone *becomes*, urging one to reorganize one's identity in order to get back on one's feet" (qtd. in Vanthuyne 413). This process of reorganising one's identity requires "illness identity work" accomplished using tools of "illness identity talk" (qtd. in Vanthuyne 413). In a way, self-representation through various discursive forms constitutes this "illness identity talk." As such, autobiographies play a major role in assisting the sufferers to find their voices and to express their idiosyncratic perceptions about living with mental illness. However, such articulation of illness experiences is not realised in isolation but is an "individualized version of a body of cultural knowledge" (413).

Crapanzano remarks how narrativisation of experience is different from passive representation:

> [It] separates the event from the flow of experience. … gives the event structure … , relates it to other similarly constructed events, and evaluates the event across both idiosyncratic and (culturally) standardized lines. Once the experience is articulated, once it is rendered an event, it is cast within the world of meaning and may then provide a basis for action.
>
> (10)

Such standardised system of values and patterns of interpretations formulates what Crapanzano refers to as a cultural idiom. These flexible codes are also appropriated by the authors in line with their experiences and specific ways of reacting to similar situations. In exploring the cultural idioms that form an inevitable part of narrating lived experiences in autobiographies, Vanthuyne identifies three types of cultural idioms that are associated with particular ways of organising the mental illness experience: the psychiatric, the emotional, and the political (423). Psychiatric idiom refers to the language specific to "biomedical epistemological views and therapeutic practices" (424) which normalise mental health problems. The emotional idiom connotes to a 'heterogeneous field of discourse' in which sufferers generate language of emotions characterised by specific personal tools that help them to cope with, as well as transcend their illness conditions (425). Addressing the limits of using emotional idiom which holds the sufferer accountable for the illness condition, the political idiom is constituted in a language which destigmatises those affected by mental illness as it "brings people to situate their mental health problems within the larger context of the social and political dynamics within which they find themselves inscribed" (426). Memoirs on the experience of mental illness combine or juxtapose each of these idioms and narrative structures which heighten subjective dimensions of patients' mental health problems, distinct from the symptomatic prescriptions in biomedical accounts.

The graphic memoirs analysed in this chapter are what Thomas Couser refers to as "nobody memoirs," for its authors are not mental health professionals and are known to the public through the publication of their illness narratives (*Memoir* 5). Introduced by Couser in his book *Memoir* to refer to photographs, paintings, and other performative arts concerned with "a discrete part of life" (23), the 'nobody memoir' has a unique democratic potential in initiating public responses towards the rights of the ill and marginalised (150).[4] For instance, Audre Lorde's *The Cancer Journals*, which raised a plethora of issues surrounding race and gender in the context of breast cancer, had a tremendous impact on the feminist movement and inaugurated new vistas of expression for those who were marginalised in multiple ways as she refused to "render invisible her difference and the experience of pain that is somehow embarrassing to others" (Zakaria). In a different way, Tamar Thembeck in her doctoral dissertation titled *Performative Autopathographies* explores the political potential of contemporary art forms like dance (Jan Bolwell's *Off My Chest,* Bill T. Jones' *Still/Here*) and photography (Jo Spence and Terry Dennett's *Property of Jo Spence?*) to delineate patients' experiences by granting their bodies a representative dimension whereby the body "becomes both a site of reception (of illness, its treatments, and its stigmatic attributions) and of active autopathographic re-inscription" (205). As such, according to Thembeck, these forms of narration enable the artists to "'survive' as an agent-subject, and to repel or rebut the silencing forces of political oppression" (200).

Like the memoirs of Lorde and others, these visual memoirs were embedded deeply in the social and engaged in challenging the dominant cultural attitudes toward illness and health and encouraging positive attitudes towards patient perspectives. For instance, several graphic memoirs like Miriam Engelberg's *Cancer Made Me a Shallower Person* and Dana Walrath's *Aliceheimer's* renegotiate and revise the dominant medical and socio-cultural scripts on cancer and Alzheimer's, respectively.[5] In illness narratives, artists often create alternative iconographies for a particular illness or refashion the existing symbols in accordance with their experiences. Either way, through dismantling negative stereotypes that surround a particular disease, these memoirs facilitate a nuanced representation of an illness condition. In their reading of *Aliceheimer's*, Sathyaraj Venkatesan and Raghavi Kasthuri demonstrate how the conscious production of a 'language of optimism' subverts the "reductive language and predictable *writing* of AD patient as brainless bodies" (79). As such, as Venkatesan and Kasthuri continue, these memoirs not only alter "the biomedical and cultural imaginaries about AD but also promise change in the experience of the patients and caregivers" by developing "the current trend of refined, affirmative, and confident representations of AD" (79–80).

To these ends, the abovementioned graphic memoirs demonstrate Margaret Price's concept of counter-diagnosis in order to explore the dynamics of illness, power, and personhood in illness narratives. Price defined counter-diagnosis as a "strategy by which those with mental disabilities use language in their autobiographies to write back to biomedical logic" (qtd. in Longhurst 40). Such counter-diagnostic complications are central to Forney's *Marbles* and Lindsay's *Rx*. In *Marbles*, Forney delineates her struggle with fluctuating moods that are characteristic of bipolar disorder and her meditations on artistic creativity and on having a diseased identity. Forney, in her quest for long-term mental stability, attempts to discover a balance of medication and lifestyle therapies, as bipolar disorder defies an easy treatment. Deploying visual metaphors and also through deftly manipulating space/page layout, Forney chronicles a range of psychic experiences from depression to manic excitement. Distancing herself from the existing discourse of mental illness as untranslatable and unavailable for representation, in *Marbles* she actualises the experience through both conventional and creative tropes. Like Forney, Lindsay also exploits the affordances of the comics medium to delineate her bipolar experience and considers her memoir *Rx* to be what Rachel Jones refers to as "a form of exorcism, a vehement statement of agency, and a necessary reckoning with her illness." The memoir represents a coming to terms with her past and present selves, while laying bare her traumatic experiences of hospitalisation. In Lindsay's terms, the memoir represents her "most authentic expression of self" ("Rachel Lindsay"). Both Forney and Lindsay, in their own terms, recast the depictions of the sufferers of mental illness by subverting the sanity/insanity binary that is prevalent in popular and medical discourses as they make their experience intelligible and available to the readers.

*Marbles* and *Rx* position themselves against codified and monotonous representations of mental illness that are available in popular and biomedical discourse as they forge a discourse of counter-diagnosis. Against this background, graphic memoirs on the experience of mental illness grant agency to sufferers to reconfigure their lived realities through strategic disorganisation and creative incoherence. Appropriating and challenging the stock patterns of medical procedures and attitudes involved in treating mental illness, these memoirs emerge as a site of productive resistance that aims to promote an alternative discourse on mental illness from patients' perspectives. Against neatly summarised and linear plot patterns of medical and popular accounts of mental illness, *Marbles* and *Rx* construct a counter-discourse where established hegemonic social codes are challenged, and domains of power are subverted through pictorial, stylistic, and spatial metaphors.

## Metaphors as Counter-Diagnostic Figurations

Predominantly through the use of metaphors, Forney and Lindsay frame their expressions of mental illness that reconfigure extant representational patterns. According to Price, these visual metaphors function as a strategy against the biomedical logic of mental illness by "subvert[ing] the diagnostic urge to 'explain' a disabled mind" (17) and by configuring the space of the comics page against what Lefebvre refers to as socially constructed spaces "of control, of domination, [and] of power" (26). In *Marbles* and in *Rx*, visual metaphors function as narratological devices with the potential to initiate such changes and to clarify abstract emotions within the narrative by relating them to other conceptual categories. The idiosyncrasies of the medium of comics justify the need for a more specific theoretical framework in terms of graphic memoirs on illness conditions, one that addresses how illness is figured not only in its written narrative, but also within the word-image interplay that is characteristic of comics. Through such stylistic drawing techniques, memoirists not only make visible their illness conditions, but also take control of the condition's aesthetics. An artist's experiential domain allows her not only to redefine her own self-perception engendered by the illness but also to expose the mainstream/dominant cultural scripts on illness that border on stigma and exclusion.

In *Marbles*, Forney illustrates several instances that reveal the overbearing influence of medical dogma over patients' perspectives. However, Forney attempts to assert herself against the homogenising medical authority of the *Diagnostic and Statistical Manual of Mental Disorders* (DSM), which is often criticised for its prescriptive symptom-based approach, which so-doing neglects psychosocial factors that also influence patients' behaviour. During the depiction of a medical appointment, Forney and the psychiatrist browse through the DSM "criteria for manic episodes" (Forney 15). Both the page composition and Forney's focalisation of the episode serve as an attempt to highlight the DSM's categorical influence. The DSM panels are composed in square frames that mimic neat and contained categorical boxes on the left side of the panel. The depiction of the DSM's straight book lines, the neat linearity of the printed text, and the psychiatrist's finger tracing a line under each symptom allegorise the medical model's linear understanding of illness.

At the form level, the panels depicting Forney's experiential understanding of each symptom contrast with the linear composition of the DSM depictions. Gradually encroaching on the space of the DSM panel, Forney's free-floating, scalloped, and amorphous balloon panel composition subverts the suggested categorical, homogenising, and linear experience of disability presented in the DSM. Forney's understanding of the diagnosis of bipolar disorder includes visual metaphors like "spinning wheels burning rubber" as the racing-mind experience of mania (17). The spinning wheels, which suggest her fast-paced thoughts, literally take the shape of her hair. In a surrealistic manner, her thoughts are spelled out across the space of the panel, and her constant chatter is signified using arrows that come out of her wide mouth. Forney's panels also constantly threaten to overlap and overtake the medical narrative of the categorical criteria of her mental illness, over the medial line of the page, and disrupt the medical panel's border, showing more favour for her experiences. Furthermore, to enhance the meaning of this visual metaphor, the artist exploits other spatial features of the comics medium, such as having a left-right orientation and a relative size. The careful positioning of the doctor's reading on the left and Forney's overcrowded balloon panel on the right align with the left-to-right reading pattern that allows readers to consider Forney's expression of the DSM with more attention. At the same time, Forney illustrates the tension by finding a middle ground between medical prescriptions of bipolarity and her experience of the same by the use of the psychiatrist having an oversized hand, in size almost equal to that of Forney's face, as depicted on the right. In a way, as Forney literally deconstructs her diagnosis of bipolar disorder through these counter-diagnostic techniques, she, as Williams points out, "enjoy[s] a modicum of power, wrestling some control away from the official arbiters of knowledge and influencing the discourse of healthcare" (par. 7).

Interestingly, Lindsay also utilises a similar stylistic technique that questions the power that is institutionalised in a way that "treats the subject of an authority as a passive recipient of the authority" (Cohen 324). The psychiatrist's oversized hand in *Marbles*, discussed above, reappears in *Rx*. In a series of silent panels, Lindsay visually demonstrates the plight of a bipolar patient who struggles to come to terms with her diagnosis and hospitalisation. Lindsay is portrayed as silently trying to escape from the panels, which crudely describe her condition in apathetic terms, into a huge blank space, while a larger-than-life hand appears on the top of the page and pinches her like a lab rat (Figure 4.1). Later, Lindsay is seen cursing and thoroughly angry at the medical system which exerts power by denying patient autonomy. In the next splash page, the hand drops her into a medical clipboard with the number 11N (Figures 4.2 and 4.3). As Lindsay explains in a lecture given at the MCPHS University, she felt "locked into a system that [she] saw no escape from" ("Rachel Lindsay"). She remarks, "now this is where I live—on that page, in that clipboard" so that she fits "someone else's definition of sanity" ("Rachel Lindsay"). Lindsay's dexterous deployment of both spatial and stylistic metaphors in these

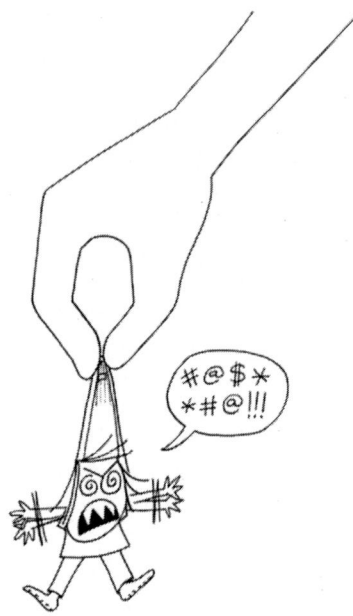

*Figure 4.1*  Lindsay being pinched up like a lab rat (*Rx*).

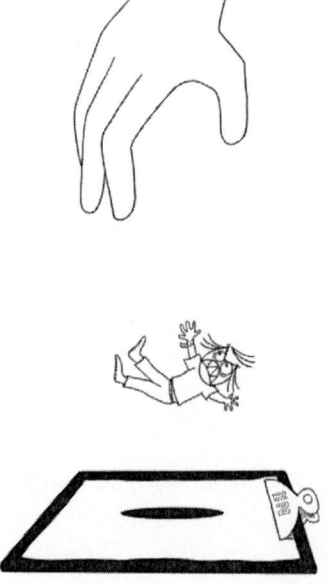

*Figure 4.2*  Lindsay being dropped into a medical chart (*Rx*).

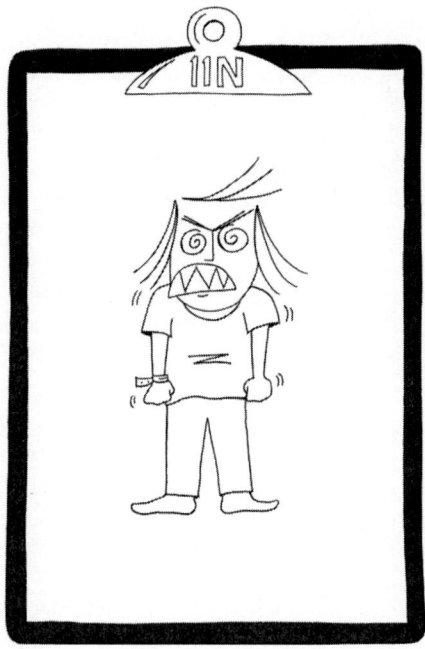

*Figure 4.3* Metaphorical representation of how Lindsay is confined to a space defined by the medical system (*Rx*).

pages serves to blatantly critique the overbearing nature of biomedical power structures that reduce people into patients with a prescribed set of observable symptoms.

Forney uses the metaphor of a carousel to illustrate the manic and depressive episodes that are characteristic of bipolar disorder. In the height of her mania, she is evidently exuberant, balancing on the horse's back. In the subsequent stages, her physiognomic features change from excitement to confusion and dismay. As such, in the depressed state she glides down from the carousel into a crouch. Here, the target of the metaphor is indicated through both words (in medical labels, such as 'hypomania,' 'euthymia,' 'dysthymia,' and 'depression') and visually. Apart from diagramming the states of bipolarity in a unique visual schema, the metaphor also economically encapsulates Forney's subjective/emotive aspects of the illness against the objective/scientific biomedical prescriptivism. Forney herself attests to the fact that "the carousel metaphor has really clarified the different mood states for [a lot of readers]" (qtd. in Klein). As the image of the carousel tends to show an association between Forney's experience of illness and such pastoral elements, it subtly displaces the rigid biomedical categorisations of bipolar diagnosis and treatment. In essence, such an attempt starkly distinguishes Forney's personal narration from the symptomatic prescriptions of biomedicine. While the DSM classifies her manic-depressive symptoms in clear statements that mimic scriptural accuracy, Forney's carousel metaphor is imbued with colloquial lexical choices and cartoon drawings that lucidly convey the nature of mood disorders for her readers.

Later, Forney improvises the carousel metaphor to a close-up segment of her heightened mania. Unlike Forney's previous blissful representation of mania, which she once thought "magical" and "vibrant" (231–232), her excitement is replaced by restlessness and compulsion. Distinct from the popular media representations of mania as a jubilant state of mind, Forney exposes the helplessness that bipolar patients experience during such uncontrollable manic episodes. Also, her deliberate choices of the carousel imagery invoke a subjective and credulous dimension of mania as being contrary the biomedical and popular representations as available in the DSM and the movies discussed above.

This episode exemplifies the way in which cross-discursiveness in comics works: visual and written narratives are juxtaposed in the structure of frames and pages, where the visual narrative delineates the character's manic mentalscape, and the written language on either side of the image signals the narrator's voice, set in the past and in the present, which are radically different in both tone and style. While the floating text on the left denotes reflections on her previous manic episodes, the regular font of the text on the right signifies the stability and balance that Forney attains through medications and alternate lifestyle practices. The page depicts three versions of the narrator's reflective present self, the manic self as the narrator's voice, and the manic past self, as represented visually. Chute refers to this characteristic of autobiographical comics as the "inbuilt duality of the form," a feature in which the "doubled narration ... visually and verbally represents the self, often in conflicting registers and different temporalities" (5). One effect from the tension arising from the conflicting discourses in comics is the denaturalisation of notions of authority in autobiography. The ontological status of the autobiographical *I* is called into question as it visually splits between a narrating *I* and a subject *I*, with the contrasting perspectives contributing to the representation of a constructed and fragmented self. In the image, the plurality of autobiographical voices is evident. Thus, in the cross-discursive function of Forney's unique carousel metaphor, the memoir verbo-visually *performs* her altered self that has evolved through a range of clinical and personal experiences. The constructedness of the memoir is exacerbated through this fragmentation of representation of the narrator's self and of her memories.

Another verbo-visual metaphor which Forney introduces captures the claustrophobia and mounting tension as she descents into depression. The metaphor spans over an entire panel where her head turns into "a cage of frantic rats" (Forney 69) that attempt to break out of her head at any moment. Pictorially and stylistically, the metaphor conveys subjective truths about being plunged into depression. The frantic rats are portrayed with hollow eyes—a visual conceit which encourages a metaphorical reading. Contrasted with Forney's wide eyes, the hollow eyes of the rats reflect the gravity of her illness condition which grind into her thoughts, devoid of any empathetic concern towards the challenges the condition forces upon Forney's life (thus deploying the conceptual metaphor, UNDERSTANDING/KNOWING IS SEEING). Thus differing from the extant representation of depression which is mostly characterised by minuscule details and stooped down face, Forney brings to the fore the initial frightening phase of depression which is absent from most popular representations. Forney's awareness of the frantic thoughts that affect her perception of head as separate from her sense of self hinges on the phenomenological notion of dys-appearance, where illness forces one's body into one's conscious awareness (El Refaie 32). The panel border is made distinct from the previous panels on the page through jagged lines, thus adding to the mounting tension and fear that Forney experiences inwardly. Here, besides representing her increasing sense of fear and unpredictability visually, the metaphor also functions as a means to negotiate the disruptions in Forney's sense of self.

The verbo-visual metaphor economically summarises Forney's subjective experience of illness by capturing the intricacies of bipolar psychic state and grants multi-layered connections to the narrative. In the previous panel, Forney contextualises the metaphor as she is shown in dire distress, calling her psychiatrist Karen for help. Here also, by carefully strewing the words 'crisis' and 'emergency' across the heavily scribbled dark background, Forney foregrounds her angst which is heightened by the apathetic automated voice from the hospital. Here, the depictions of fear and distress that accompanies depression, unlike popular representations, are not limited to the patient's worried facial expression and frightened eyes. In the succeeding verbo-visual metaphor, the readers are exposed to the intensity with which depression impacts the patient in an affective way. At three distinct levels, the metaphor communicates the author's mental landscape—the narrating *I* in the text box ("my head was a cage of frantic rats") presents the metaphor clearly; the subject *I* in speech balloon, "Karen! I'm scared," denotes an element of fear which is absent in the statement of the narrating *I*; and the autobiographical *I* visually depicts the contours of Forney's frightening descent into depression through her wide, staring eyes, the ferocious group of rats stuck in her head, and the jagged panel border which simulates the rats' sharp teeth.

## Deconstructing Stereotypes

As many popular and medical representations presume violence and abnormal behaviour as the characteristic symptoms of mental illness, the mentally ill suffer exclusion from mainstream society. Like Forney, Lindsay also expresses her rage and anxiety in the face of stigma of her illness condition. The fear of social exclusion that Lindsay experiences is metaphorically portrayed both visually and verbally (Figure 4.4), in that she visually embodies herself as a wolf with blank eyes and a grim expression. Such an anthropomorphic attribute is reminiscent of Spiegelman's *Maus,* in which he recounts the horrors of the Holocaust by portraying the Jews as mice and the Nazis as cats. Lindsay uses a similar predator-prey relationship to foreground the social antagonism towards the mentally ill who are denigrated as violent and

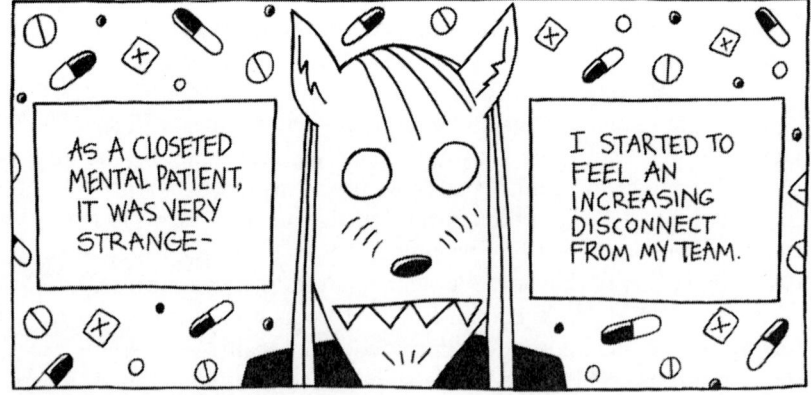

*Figure 4.4* Lindsay's self-representation as a wolf (*Rx*).

dangerous. As such, Lindsay's wolf avatar signifies her internalised fears of being stigmatised. In a radio interview with Jane Lindholm, Lindsay remarks that the wolf is "a powerful visual for the 'dangerous' creature that was within [her]self." While the subject *I* of the autobiographical self is visually depicted through Lindsay's external wolf-like features that suggest her inner fears caused by 'otherness,' the narrating *I* in the text boxes expresses her increasing sense of disconnect and denotes shame and stigma.

The panel background is patterned with tablets and capsules of various shapes and sizes, signifying the pressure of being medicated to remain 'sane.' This verbo-visual metaphor at once comments on the existing social status of a person diagnosed with mental illness, specifically bipolar disorder, as well as its impact on the patient whose identity is no different from that of a banished wolf.

Lindsay improvises the metaphor of the wolf in several episodes in the memoir. In the third chapter, titled "Passing," the plot steers towards Lindsay's successful career as she gets promoted to a Pfizer account executive. The splash page portrays Lindsay as a wolf in sheep's clothing as she shifts to her new office, while the other employees are portrayed as sheep. As the title of the chapter suggests, Lindsay had to be extremely careful in the way she carried herself as she was always subjected to the scrutiny of those who only approved of what is 'normal.' In her interview with Lindholm, Lindsay confesses that she "didn't feel comfortable at all with anyone knowing that [she] was bipolar" and that if she were to reveal that she had a mood disorder, she wouldn't be "trusted with managing the client's money." Regarding the particular episode, Lindsay herself attests to a "strong sense of 'otherness'" that she experienced and an increasing sense of "self-stigma and self-hatred" that she harboured within in comparison to her "normal" peers (Lindholm).

The metaphor of the wolf in sheep's clothing further hints at the way society regards the mentally ill as being pretentious and hypocritical (Howard). Presumed to be irresponsible and uncontrollable, mentally ill are often excluded and humiliated. Because of this, the immense pressure of acting like an 'ordinary' and 'sane' individual is clearly laid out elsewhere when Lindsay is brought to her knees in the workplace staring at her desktop while the background depicts capsules and tablets that rain over her. The text box in the panel, "whose life was I actually living," echoes throughout the episode as she struggles to maintain her 'sane,' sheep-like appearance to remain aligned with her professional space. After a series of such debilitating episodes, Lindsay depicts herself as a wolf, erasing her external features (like her straight long hair), exhausted in front of her desktop under a spot-light. In this situation, the metaphor of the wolf, which develops in subsequent stages in the memoir, effectively captures her predicament as someone who has bipolar disorder and who is forced to suffer exclusion if he or she doesn't meet the tenets of 'normalcy.' As Lindsay explains in an interview with Jones, drawing different versions of her avatar "has helped [her] to conceive of toxic selves, recognize when they come up and separate them from [her] actual self." Her need to stay sane, however, lands her in a cyclical conundrum of medication, health insurance, and employment.

As Lindsay remarks in the first chapter of *Rx*, preconceived standards of the sanity/insanity binary inevitably force one to strive towards a 'single, somber objective' of 'staying sane' and abhor divergent behavioural patterns that deflect from "normalcy" (*Rx*). In this context, Lindsay dexterously exposes the constructed nature of sanity/insanity through a poster representing the physical attributes of a 'sane' individual (Figure 4.5). An emotionless and sombre face drawn in clear simple lines is suspended between the words 'staying' and 'sane' in the

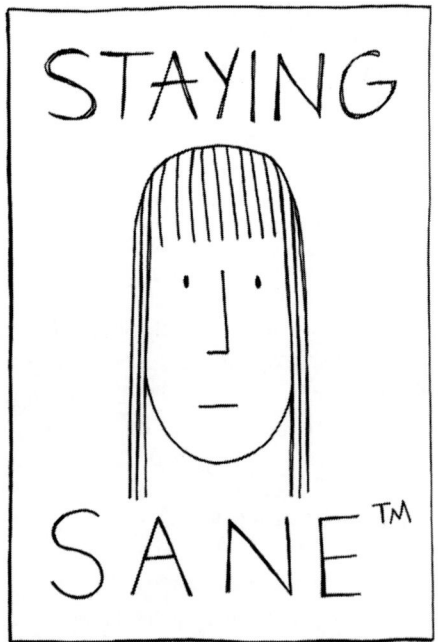

*Figure 4.5* The sanity poster (*Rx*).

poster. In a way, Lindsay mimics the logic of visual representations of mental illness, which very often portray symptomatic features of bipolar disorder in stock images. Accordingly, the poster performs an alternative function aimed at busting the notions of in/sanity by literalising the presumed notions of rationality.

Elsewhere, Lindsay lashes out at the socio-cultural and biomedical systems that constantly monitor one's behaviour for signs of sanity/insanity through a compelling verbo-visual metaphor (Figure 4.6). Lindsay portrays herself as a performer, tapping her feet and dancing with a cane and hat in her hospital gown and name tag. Although Lindsay appears jubilant, the visual details and the caption ("in a lot of ways, sanity is a performance") at once present a grim reality of the world that Lindsay, as a bipolar patient, inhabits as it deconstructs the insanity/sanity binary. While the stage, spotlight, and the audience, which belong to the conceptual category of performances, serve as the source domain of the verbo-visual metaphor, the caption anchors it to the conceptual category of sanity/insanity, which is the target domain. Lindsay portrays herself in the first panel with the audience drawn in shadows. In the subsequent panel, the readers encounter the audience who are comprised of bespectacled doctors/psychiatrists busily taking notes on Lindsay's behaviour. Interestingly, the image of the doctors who are portrayed with spectacles over hollow eyes is based on a conceptual metaphor—UNDERSTANDING/ KNOWING IS SEEING—to connote the indifference of medical professionals who are blind to their patients' perspectives. That is to say that these doctors are indifferent to Lindsay's bipolar condition, and through constant monitoring, they belittle the patient's dignity. Here, unlike popular representations of mental illness and mental asylums, which accentuate patients' postures from crude angles, Lindsay exposes the monotony that pervades clinical settings and the striking apathy of medical professionals towards the mentally ill. The image also succinctly captures an episode of depersonalising the mentally ill under the medical system's behest, although the medical system is meant to serve for their rehabilitation and recovery.

In a distinct vein, the caption, "sanity is a performance," questions the standardised logic of insanity and the consequent exclusion that the mentally ill suffer. The caption draws together the sanity poster and the wolf-sheep episodes in a subversive light in order to illustrate how sane appearances and the stock images of insanity are merely roles that are fashioned by popular and medical discourses. Thus, the different roles that each individual assumes by repetitive action are not intrinsic to an individual's identity but are constituted, as Foucault

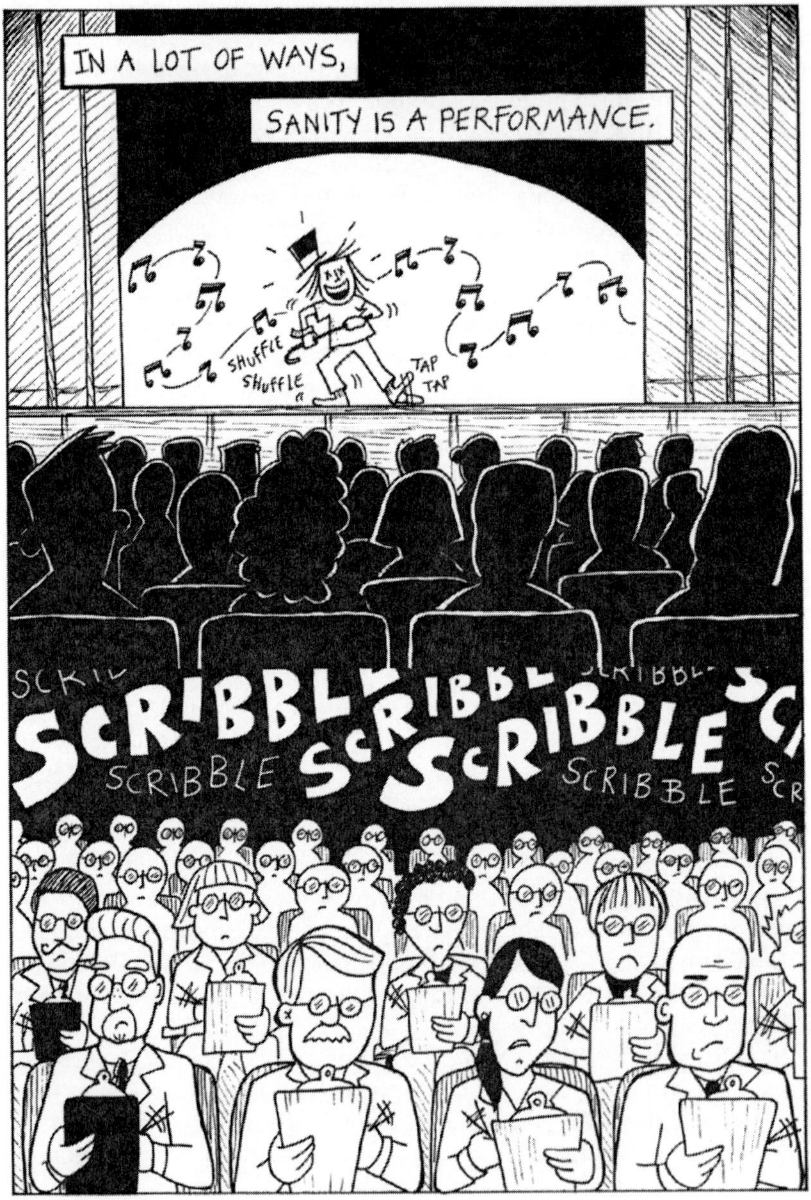

*Figure 4.6* Sanity as performance (*Rx*).

remarks, through performances of language, gestures, and signs that are mediated by social agents (qtd. in Young). These social agents constitute a discourse of mental illness and exercise power by enforcing norms of what is rational, sane, or true. However, Foucault argues that these discourses are not subservient to power but can be used as "a point of resistance and a starting point for an opposing strategy" (101). Lindsay's visual metaphor of insanity/sanity performance not only exposes medical professionals as the agents who constitute the norms of sanity but also becomes an opposing strategy that counters such diagnostic logic by equating sanity and insanity in a verbo-visual schema.

Also, by stating that sanity is a performance, Lindsay adheres to the Butlerian notion of performativity as an "act that one performs, [which] is, in a sense, an act that has been going on before one arrived on the scene" (Butler 526). Butler also argues that such performances that lead to subject formation have to be "cultivated, policed, and enforced; and the violation of that has to be punished, usually through shame" (Kotz). In this light, one can see Lindsay as subverting the sanity/insanity binary through the verbo-visual metaphor that re-enacts such policed and enforced behaviours that are grouped into either of these categories.

Deliberately unsettling the fixity of the binary opposition sanity/insanity, Lindsay forges a new theoretical space that demands a redefinition of the rigid categorisations of opposites. Put differently, Lindsay's statement, "sanity is a performance," and her deft use the visual metaphor not only allows the readers to "see a mentally ill individual as more than her illness" but also "challenges the binary structure of thought that underlies categorizing human beings as sick or healthy, able or disabled" (Sherman 166). When sanity is deemed as performance, boundaries between the sane and insane are blurred and the forces which create those boundaries are equally exposed. To this end, *Rx* demands a paradigm shift in order to recognise the socio-cultural and biomedical forces that draft such rigid demarcations between sane and insane patterns that lead to the depersonalisation of the mentally ill. In so doing, Lindsay's metaphor represent a continuum where sanity and insanity are constructed and assigned to select individuals by institutional power structures rather than as two mutually exclusive states of mind.

## Conclusion

Apart from the travails of the illnesses that patients suffer from, the mentally ill are doubly challenged by the stereotypes that ensue from misconceptions about mental illness in popular media and medical discourse. As such, representations that negatively portray the mentally ill also shape caregivers' perspectives towards mental illness. Generalised and unscientific assumptions about the illness could cause caregivers to disregard patients' individuality or the distinct nature of the illness. Adding to such familial neglect, the social life of the mentally ill are also adversely affected. Specifically, according to Corrigan and Watson, in policy-making and in resource allocation, the mentally ill are denied opportunities required for quality living, ranging from satisfactory jobs and healthcare facilities, to affiliations with a diverse group of people (35).

In this context, the personal accounts of illness experience develop a parallel alternate discourse about what it means to live with mental illness by challenging the extant stereotypes in popular media, public discourse, and other forms of cultural and biological reductionism. Similarly, a movement away from categories of symptoms and signs, in a way, fosters creative and novel representations of mental illness experiences and the complexities of an altered internal reality. Graphic memoirs, as the ones discussed in this chapter, stimulate a rethinking of mental illness as a singular experience as they "create a linguistic, co-created place for transactions and translations between patients [and] medical specialists" (Kristeva et al. 57) and the public in visually engaging ways. In effect, these memoirs on bipolar disorder aim to problematise the politics of representations pertaining to the mentally ill by laying bare the stigmatising and exclusionary nature of such imaginings.

These discussions acknowledge the questions posed at the beginning of this chapter. Graphic memoirs such as *Marbles* and *Rx* counterweigh the iconographic control of biomedical and popular discourses. Against such biomedical models that attempt to normalise, homogenise, and pathologise mental conditions, Forney and Lindsay particularise and individualise their experiences in *Marbles* and *Rx,* respectively, which according to Couser is synonymous with *"owning diagnosis"* ("Is There" 19). As such, the comics medium grants the artists greater control in representing their self-image. At the intersection of text and image, the author/artist reveals simultaneously what is explicitly spoken and subtly suggested. Unlike medical illustrations, according to Williams, comics do not claim verisimilitude nor accuracy while utilising a range of rhetorical visual devices like metaphors, humour, and abstractions "to articulate the feelings associated with the illness, offering a window into their subjective realities" (par. 10). Forney and Lindsay deploy specific techniques that invite the *mind* into the narrative in distinct ways, both literally and metaphorically. Such spatial and stylistic techniques engender a constructive unsettling that prompts readers to take a more informed stance towards illness. In deploying metaphorical expressions which capture their unique mental experiences, these authors deconstruct the harmful and limited binaries of sanity and insanity. In so doing, they regain control over representation of their self-image. Consequently, according to Thembeck, the authors of these graphic memoirs and the community of sufferers that they constitute through identification "become active agents in their personal, political, and cultural negotiations of health and disease" (275).

The multimodal space of comics coupled with its unique affordances enables autobiographical subjects to represent themselves in multiple ways, challenging singular or static modes of self-representation. As discussed in this chapter, both Forney and Lindsay deconstruct the prescribed notions of mental illness by juxtaposing standardised diagnostic manuals like the DSM and an alternate representation of the symptoms from a subjective position. Utilising tools of counter-diagnosis like verbo-visual metaphors, their memoirs evolve as a counter-space where subjective and emotional truths gather momentum over the biomedical and popular discourses of mastery. Comics also provide a safe space for author and reader alike to examine this oscillation between standardised representative modes and identity constructions through cross-discursive patterns that verbo-visual metaphors entail. By including varied embodiments of illness conditions through such multiple modes of representation, these memoirs pluralise the self-representation of illness, countering the singular view of normalcy that relies on monotony, and thus, they humanise mental illness. Such diverse representations of mental illness in graphic memoirs as these challenges the homogeneous expectation implied by the normalising standards set by popular and biomedical representations. In practical terms, such subversions and revisions grafted into the discourse on mental illness via graphic memoirs expose the depersonalising episodes rampant within clinical settings. In the context of *Marbles* and *Rx*, readers (be they healthcare professionals or laypersons) are demanded to think about mental illness beyond stereotypes with nuance and complexity. Graphic memoirs thus reconstitute a lost sense of identity that need not comply with the neat and linear structures of canonical genres.

## Acknowledgement

This chapter is derived in part from an article published in the *Journal of Graphic Novels and Comics* on 11 July 2019 © Taylor & Francis, available online: https://doi.org/10.1080/21504857.2019.1641531.

## Notes

1 According to the United States National Institute of Mental Health, bipolar disorder is "a mental disorder that causes unusual shifts in mood, energy, activity levels, concentration, and the ability to carry out day-to-day tasks." ("Bipolar Disorder." *National Institute of Mental Health,* January 2020, https://www.nimh.nih.gov/health/topics/bipolar-disorder/index.shtml.)
2 Over 500 comments to the short film, "Bipolar" uploaded to YouTube attests to the viewer's protest against the inaccurate portrayals of bipolar disorder. Here are two examples:

> The person who made this short film doesn't understand Bipolar.
>
> (Safira Fitri)

> I am glad I'm not the only one who most deff agree this is not bipolar. I have no idea what I just saw.
>
> (Xico Alva)

3 Malayalam movies are produced in the state of Kerala, India. The official language is Malayalam. Besides *Vadakkunnathan,* several other movies like *Thalavattam* (1986), *Thaniyavarthanam* (1987), *Aham* (1992), and *Manichithrathazhu* (1993) portray mental illness. (See K. V. Menon and Ranjith, G. "Malayalam Cinema and Mental Health.")
4 In *Memoir,* Couser alludes to movements like the Gay Rights movement and Disability Rights movement in the United States which were inspired by "nobody memoirs" (150).
5 See Venkatesan and Kasthuri. "'Magic and Laughter': Graphic Medicine, Recasting Alzheimer Narratives and Dana Walrath's *Aliceheimer's: Alzheimer's Through the Looking Glass.*"

## Reference List

"Bipolar || Short Film." *YouTube,* uploaded by reduxproductions, 17 October 2013, https://www.youtube.com/watch?v=negr4U79PUE.

Boysen, Guy A., et al. "Evidence for Blatant Dehumanization of Mental Illness and its Relation to Stigma." *The Journal of Social Psychology,* vol. 160, no. 3, 2019, pp. 346–356. doi: 10.1080/00224545.2019.1671301.

Butler, Judith. "Performative Acts and Gender Constitution: An Essay in Phenomenology and Feminist Theory." *Theatre Journal,* vol. 40, no. 4, 1988, pp. 519–531. doi: 10.2307/3207893.

Chute, Hillary. *Graphic Women: Life Narrative and Contemporary Comics.* Columbia UP, 2010.

Cohen, Elliot D. *Critical Thinking Unleashed.* Rowman & Littlefield, 2009.

Corrigan, Patrick W., and Amy C. Watson. "The Paradox of Self-Stigma and Mental Illness." *Clinical Psychology: Science and Practice,* vol. 9, no. 1, 2002, pp. 35–53.

Couser, Thomas G. "Is There a Body in This Text? Embodiment in Graphic Somatography." a/b: *Auto/Biography Studies.* Advance online publication, 2018, doi: 10.1080/08989575.2018.1445585.

———. *Memoir: An Introduction.* Oxford UP, 2012.

Crapanzano, Vincent. "Introduction." *Case Studies in Spirit Possession,* edited by Vincent Crapanzano and Vivian Garrison, John Wiley and Sons, 1977, pp. 1–40.

El Refaie, Elisabeth. *Visual Metaphor and Embodiment in Graphic Illness Narratives.* Oxford UP, 2019.

Felman, Shoshana. *Writing and Madness.* Stanford UP, 2003.

Forney, Ellen. *Marbles: Mania, Depression, Michelangelo, &Me: A Graphic Memoir.* Penguin, 2012.

Foucault, Michel. *The History of Sexuality: An Introduction,* translated by R. Hurley. Penguin, 1990.

Gilmore, Leigh. *Autobiographics: A Feminist Theory of Women's Self Representation.* Cornell UP, 1994.

Howard, Gabe. "I Have Bipolar and Anxiety Disorder and I'm a Hypocrite." *GabeHoward,* 21 January 2017, http://www.gabehoward.com/bipolar-anxiety-disorder-im-hypocrite/.

Jones, Rachel E. "Rachel Lindsay's Graphic Memoir 'Rx' Creates a Buzz." *Vermont's Independent Voice,* 5 September 2018, https://www.sevendaysvt.com/vermont/rachel-lindsays-graphic-memoir-rx-creates-a-buzz/Content?oid=20063496.

Klein, Sarah. "What Bipolar Disorder Really Feels Like." *HuffPost,* 18 September 2014, https://www.huffingtonpost.in/2014/09/18/bipolar-disorder-ellen-forney_n_5823138.html.

Kotz, Liz. "The Body You Want: Liz Kotz Interviews Judith Butler." *Artforum,* vol. 31, no. 3, 1992, pp. 82–89.

Kristeva, Julia, et al. "Cultural Crossings of Care: An Appeal to the Medical Humanities." *Med Humanit,* no. 44, 2018, pp. 55–58. doi: 10.1136/medhum-2017–011263.

Lefebvre, Henri. *The Production of Space,* translated by D. Nicholson-Smith. Basil Blackwell, 1991.

Lindholm, Jane. "'RX': Cartoonist Rachel Lindsay's Tale of Living with Bipolar Disorder." *VPR,* 31 August 2018, https://www.vpr.org/post/rx-cartoonist-rachellindsays-tale-living-bipolar-disorder.

Lindsay, Rachel. *Rx: A Graphic Memoir.* Grand Central, 2018.

Longhurst, Katrina. "Counterdiagnosis and the Critical Medical Humanities: Reading Susanna Kaysen's *Girl, Interrupted* and Lauren Slater's *Lying: A Metaphorical Memoir.*" *Medical Humanities,* vol. 47, no. 1, 2021, pp. 38–46.

Menon, Koravangattu V., and Gopinath Ranjith. "Malayalam Cinema and Mental Health." *International Review of Psychiatry,* vol. 21, no. 3, 2009, pp. 218–223.

O'Hern, Declan. "An Analysis of Bipolar Disorder Stereotypes in Television Programming." *Elon Journal of Undergraduate Research in Communications,* vol. 8, no. 2, 2017, pp. 67–76.

Price, Margaret. "Her Pronouns Wax and Wane": Psychosocial Disability, Autobiography, and Counter-Diagnosis. *Journal of Literary & Cultural Disability Studies,* vol. 3, 2009, pp. 11–33.

"Rachel Lindsay Reclaiming the Patient Narrative in Graphic Medicine." *YouTube*, uploaded by MK Czerwiec, 15 April 2019, https://www.youtube.com/watch?v=VK_BJwCQFUE.

Ratnakaran, B., et al. "Psychiatric Disorders in Malayalam Cinema." *Kerala Journal of Psychiatry*, vol. 28, no. 2, 2015, http://kjponline.com/index.php/kjp/article/view/52/pdf.

Sherman, Gail Berkeley. "'My Difference Is Not My [Mental] Sickness': Ethnicity and Erasure in Joanne Greenberg's Jewish American Life Writing." *Literatures of Madness: Disability Studies and Mental Health*, edited by Elizabeth J. Donaldson, Palgrave MacMillan, 2018, pp. 165–182.

Smith, Sidonie, and Julia Watson. *Reading Autobiography: A Guide for Interpreting Life Narratives*. U of Minnesota P, 2001.

"11 Superheroes with Bipolar Disorder." *Blahpolar*, 30 July 2015, https://theblahpolar.wordpress.com/2015/07/30/10-superheroes-with-bipolar-disorder/.

Thembeck, Tamar. *Performative Autopathographies: Self-Representations of Physical Illness in Contemporary Art*. 2009. McGill U. PhD dissertation.

Vann, Madeline R. "Are People with Bipolar Disorder Dangerous?" *Everyday Health*, 13 July 2010, https://www.everydayhealth.com/bipolar-disorder/are-people-with-bipolar-disorder-dangerous.aspx.

Vanthuyne, Karine. "Searching for the Words to Say It: The Importance of Cultural Idioms in the Articulation of the Experience of Mental Illness." *Ethos*, vol. 31, no. 3, 2003, pp. 412–433.

Venkatesan, Sathyaraj, and Raghavi Ravi Kasthuri. ""Magic and Laughter": Graphic Medicine, Recasting Alzheimer Narratives and Dana Walrath's Aliceheimer's: Alzheimer's through the Looking Glass." *Concentric: Literary and Cultural Studies*, vol. 44, no. 1, 2018, pp. 61–84.

Williams, Ian. "The Iconography of Illness and Suffering in Graphic Pathographies." *Comics and Medicine Conference* Toronto, 24 July 2012. PDF File.

Wiltshire, John. "Biography, Pathography, and the Recovery of Meaning." *The Cambridge Quarterly*, vol. 29, no. 4, 2000, pp. 409–422.

Young, Stephen. "Judith Butler: Performativity." *Critical Legal Thinking*, 14 November 2016, http://criticallegalthinking.com/2016/11/14/judith-butlers-performativity/.

Zakaria, Rafia. "The Cancer Journals Record a New Way for Women to Face Ill-health." *The Guardian*, 30 December 2016, https://www.theguardian.com/books/booksblog/2016/dec/30/the-cancer-journals-record-a-new-way-for-women-to-face-ill-health.

# 5 Visual Metaphors of OCD and Schizophrenia

## Introduction

Various medium-specific elements of comics enable artists/patients who suffer from mental illnesses to approximate their experiential reality via graphic narratives. The fictional narratives analysed in this chapter, *Swallow Me Whole* and *The Nao of Brown*, are reflections of Nate Powell's and Glyn Dillon's experiences of dealing with friends and family members who suffer from mental conditions such as obsessive compulsive disorder (OCD) and schizophrenia. Weaving together dreams, myths, and reality, Powell and Dillon create complex narratives that bring to life the patients' subjective worlds. In so doing, these narratives negotiate an alternate reality which is not captured in biomedical and popular accounts of the illness conditions. Spatial and stylistic visual metaphors are used in these narratives to depict specific psychological experiences in viscerally engaging ways. Drawing theoretical insights from El Refaie and S. Kay Toombs, this chapter aims to explore the middle ground between triumphalist and fatalist narratives through visual metaphors that stylistically encapsulate the patient's lived experience. It also investigates how Nate Powell's *Swallow Me Whole* (2008) and Glyn Dillon's *The Nao of Brown* (2012) use stylistic and spatial metaphors to intersperse multiple temporal and spatial dimensions that mimic patient's altered inner world.

## Perspectives in Context

Patients diagnosed with psychiatric disorders such as schizophrenia are approached with caution and often stereotyped as violent and dangerous (See Chapter 3). OCD is sometimes misdiagnosed and regarded by the patients themselves as simply a dimension of their personality, whereas people diagnosed with schizophrenia are considered

DOI: 10.4324/9781003214229-6

"unpredictable and incompetent" (Angermeyer and Matschinger 1049). In both cases, patients' experiences are under-represented, which forces them to navigate their alternate psychic worlds on their own. Most clinical encounters fail to address these issues, as the physician presumes a dominant status in the clinical setting. In *Narrative Medicine*, Charon argues that physicians need "empathy, humility, trustworthiness and respect" (4) to engage effectively with patients. A doctor's failure or disinterest in addressing a patient's emotional landscape often leads to marginalisation. If clinical encounters were characterised by empathetic interactions, they would alleviate the emotional and social pressures that shape patients' experience of their illness. Appropriate and timely communication about the risks and benefits of an illness results in trust between doctor and patient, and also prepares the patient to confront his or her illness effectively. Furthermore, a doctor/caregiver who approaches a patient suffering from OCD or schizophrenia with empathy helps alleviate the stigma associated with the illness.

OCD is clinically defined by the presence of obsessions and compulsions which are "excessive or unreasonable, and [...] cause marked distress, are time consuming, or significantly interfere with the patients functioning" (Hudak and Dougherty 1). In their book *Obsessive Compulsive Disorder*, Naomi A. Fineberg and Dan J. Stein define OCD as "characterised by intrusive, unpleasant thoughts or images (obsessions), and by repetitive, unwanted actions (compulsions) that are performed in response to obsessions or according to rigid rules" (5). Several other studies have observed that the sufferers of OCD cannot control their obsessive thoughts and compulsive practices (Baer 7; Fileva 285; Tompkins 10). Most patients who suffer from OCD refuse to seek help or share the "bizarre nature of [their] obsessive thoughts" and consequently experience "shame, fear, and denial" (Tompkins 3) in social situations. While the clinical definition of schizophrenia has evolved over the centuries, most recent resources characterise it as a "serious psychiatric disorder with [a] heterogeneous symptoms profile characterised by the presence of positive and negative symptoms, such as agitation, hallucinations, delusions, and lack of emotion" (Arozal et al. 57). Several others regard it as a "disintegration of the self," manifesting as "'splitting of the psyche' or 'loosening of associations'" (Postmes et al. 41–42), which induces hallucinations and delusions in the sufferer. People with schizophrenia are often considered to be "more dangerous, aggressive [and] prone to crime" (Yılmaz et al. 297), and hence suffer "high rates of unemployment and a reduced life expectancy" (Li et al. 225). Owing to these vulnerabilities and over-generalised clinical labels inclined towards lack of reason or emotion, patients are often discriminated against in diverse spheres of life. Graphic novels such as Nate Powell's *Swallow Me Whole* and Glyn Dillon's *The Nao of Brown* emerge as significant alternatives to the prevailing clinical and popular perspectives on schizophrenia and OCD, respectively. In delineating the nuances of the protagonists' inner reality, these narratives compel the reader to experience the alternate world perceived by the patients themselves and thus counter popular notions that these illnesses are characterised by violence or incoherence.

Apart from these graphic narratives, Clem and Olivier Martini's graphic memoir *Bitter Medicine: A Graphic Memoir of Mental Illness* (2010) and Von Allan's graphic novel *The Road to God Knows* (2009) also chronicle the tribulations of schizophrenia and related mental illness conditions. Graphic memoirs such as Jason Adam Katzenstein's *Everything Is an Emergency: An OCD Story in Words & Pictures* (2020), John Porcellino's *The Hospital Suite* (2014), and Adam Bourret's *I'm Crazy* (2009) visualise OCD experiences. On the other hand, Lily Williams's web comics details her "O.C.D. Story" using rich visual metaphors. The speech balloons, for instance, that echo her inner fears are shaped like flames of fire that constantly threaten her existence as she walks through a dark and narrow pathway of uncertainty. Each comic page on the screen thus simultaneously presents her struggles and ways of coping with them using various verbo-visual techniques. Williams also provides links to online resources that help readers understand the nuances of OCD and seek clinical support if required. While these narratives include autobiographical and fictional accounts of patients suffering from the OCD, Williams' *The Bad Doctor: The Troubled Life and Times of Dr. Iwan James* (2014) is a semi-autobiographical narrative from the distinct perspective of a health professional who dares to present his vulnerabilities (as opposed to the popular toxic macho ideals of a doctor). Accentuated by symbolism and black humour, Williams delves into the character's personal and professional life which is tinted and shaped by his OCD past. The frequent flashbacks of his childhood mental rituals invite the readers into an alternate space where visual metaphors of his turbulent psychogeography are stylised with rich gradients of black and white. These graphic narratives, thus, replace stereotypes about mental illnesses such as schizophrenia and OCD with personal and genuine expressions of fear bordering on a desire to overcome the perils of stigma. Steering away from monolithic voices of biomedicine, graphic medicine espouses these narratives with such rich and varied perspectives.

Powell's *Swallow Me Whole*, which was published in 2008 by Top Shelf, revolves around the world of two step-siblings, Ruth and Perry, who suffer from schizophrenia. Perry hallucinates a "little wizard" which forces him to draw incessantly, whereas Ruth sees a plethora of insects and other mysterious creatures which force their way into her room through windows and ventilation slits. Powell effortlessly inter-weaves their hallucinations and the ordinary events of their lives in the narrative, thus capturing the realistic nature of their mental landscapes and making the narrative compelling. Both Perry and Ruth experience intriguing visions that no one else sees. Powell invites the reader into their unique worlds through stylistic visual images and metaphors. Although *Swallow Me Whole* is a work of fiction, Powell himself has said that the main themes, such as familial history of illness and fasci-nation with insects, are drawn from his personal life. In an interview with *ComicMix*, Powell talked about several links between the narra-tive and significant events from his own life:

> my three surviving grandparents died in spring of 2004, and much of the book was a product of wading through that. For the last decade I've worked for folks with developmental disabilities, and a lot of mental health issues go hand-in-hand.
>
> (Troup)

Powell also remarks that a large part of his life was "spent around and in support of people who have trouble navigating through a rigid world, who have wildly different perspectives and cognitive styles" (Troup).

Published in 2012 by Self Made Hero, Dillon's *The Nao of Brown*, on the other hand, tells the story of a *hafu* (half-Japanese, half-English) girl, Nao, who suffers from OCD. Nao struggles to control her violent urges to harm those who are weaker than her. She is also obsessed with a Japanese comic called *ichi* and falls in love with a washing machine repairman who looks like one of the characters in *ichi*. Their conversa-tions and Nao's experiences at the Buddhist meditation centre revolve around life philosophies which defy easy categorisation into good and bad. In one sense Dillon is examining how a binary approach to good and bad becomes the main cause of Nao's obsessive and com-pulsive thought patterns; however, Dillon deconstructs the binary by interspersing Nao's story with a plot from a Japanese manga series, *ichi*, that has striking parallels with Nao's own life. Similarities in plot apart, the narratives differ substantively in drawing and narrative style. The story of the *ichi* character Pictor evokes surreal and fantastic elements without speech or thought balloons, whereas Nao's narrative is both visually and verbally explicit about her inner feelings and thoughts. Pictor's narrative is carefully interwoven with Nao's story in such a way that it mimics the complex nature of Nao's obsessions and compulsions. The binary of good and bad and her conflicted identity as a half-Japanese person are deconstructed in the final lines of the Pictor narrative as Nao reconciles, thus: "Brown or black and white, /I then became all Nothing, /And day was wed with night" (Dillon 190).

## Picturing the Psychicscape through Spatial and Stylistic Metaphors

Both Powell and Dillon converge the patient's internal and external realities through metaphorical representations. Visual metaphors that are based on bodily experience "in space and in relation to other people, creatures, and objects" (El Refaie 85) are called spatial metaphors, whereas stylistic metaphors "use formal features such as brightness, colour, form, level of detail, and quality of line, as well as actual or implied material qualities of the page or the whole book, to indicate an abstract concept or a non-visual sense perception" (El Refaie 86). Both spatial and stylistic metaphors play a crucial role in externalising the complex nature of schizophrenic minds, which are characterised by "uncontrollable, parallel trains of thoughts, occurring simultaneously with a loss of meaning, and experiences of sudden, complete emptiness of thoughts" (Parnas and Henriksen 77). The patient's experiences in real and imagined spaces correspond to the two spatial levels employed in comics, namely the "space of the story world" and the "space of the page" (El Refaie 103). By using multiple spatial dimensions the artist is able to depict the alternate realities experienced by the patient truthfully.

Echoing the theoretical propositions of conceptual metaphor theory (CMT), conceptual metaphors such as IDEAL IS UP/REAL IS DOWN; UNREALISTIC IS UP are represented spatially in the medium of comics, by placing the hallucinations and fantasies that accompany schizophrenia at the top of a page or floating across the panels. El Refaie has commented that in most mental illness narratives, UP is "frequently associated with mental processes, dreams, fantasies, and illusions, which when they are represented visually, are almost invariably positioned above the character's heads" (103). Such metaphorical representations could be inspired by bodily experiences as proposed in CMT. For instance, the positioning of dreams and fantasies at the top of the page of a comic is based on the fact that the human brain in located at the top of the body (El Refaie 104). Both Powell and Dillon experiment with the spatial dimensions of comics in their representation of the mental landscape of characters who suffer from schizophrenia and OCD. Powell, for instance, represents onomatopoeic words in pictures which spill over panel and page boundaries to convey their tremendous impact on the protagonist, who is occasionally haunted by the voices she hears (Figure 5.1). These panels could be referred to as "mental-space evoking panels" (Cohn 81) which evoke "larger semantic frames or connect mental spaces" of the storyworld and the protagonist's psychic experience to create conceptual metaphors (81). Although the characters and objects remain within the panel boundaries, magical creatures and their voices are illustrated across the full area of the page, flying in and out of panels and gutters to suggest the threatening nature of hallucinations. In other words, this metaphorical framework implies unseen events from Ruth's imaginary world which is embedded into the visual morphology of the text. A particular feature of Powell's work is the use of such spatial metaphors constituted with hallucinatory images and words always flowing to the right, thus signifying their persistent nature.

El Refaie remarks that drawing style is "an expression of an artist's unique personality and perspective" (109). Several other scholars, including Carney, Chaney, and Miodrag, have made similar observations and suggested that stylistic metaphors enable readers to "see the world through one of the character's eyes and/or to emphasise key themes" (El Refaie 109). Dillon's memoir is replete with stylistic metaphors that convey the protagonist's intense struggle with her thoughts, which she describes thus: "awful thoughts ... that just hit me ... yesss, hit me like a fucking hammer to my head" (165). Although Dillon often maintains the traditional grid pattern (3×3) in the memoir, Nao's psychic turmoil is brought to life in the diverse shades of red used to distinguish her violent thoughts from the real events that are illustrated elsewhere. The attire of the characters and the panel backgrounds are predominantly represented in deep red shades during episodes where the protagonist, who suffers from OCD, experiences uncontrollable emotions that spill over into frustrated gestures and body postures. Although such use of colour is often considered symbolic rather than metaphorical, El Refaie argues that human response to colour is 'deeply embodied' and therefore in certain contexts, colours act as metaphors for particular emotions and physiological traits (112). For instance, since red is the colour with the longest wavelength and lowest frequency, it remains on photoreceptors of the eye for longest, hence its association with danger; moreover, red is associated with violence and excitement because

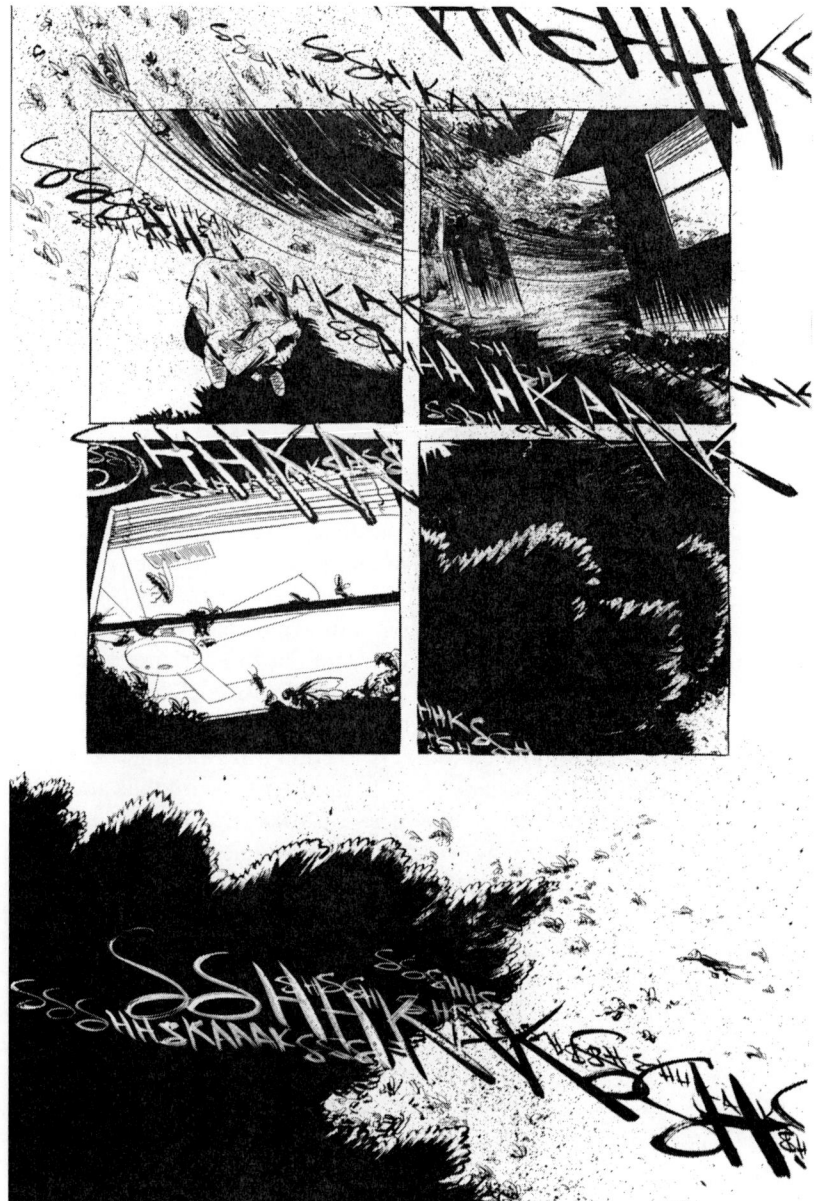

*Figure 5.1* Ruth's hallucinations (*Swallow Me Whole*).

red is the colour of blood (El Refaie 112). Dillon also preserves the colour motif in the materiality of the book by shading its fore edge in red, which metaphorically signifies Nao's obsessive mental condition. As Wolk argues, stylistic choices about the materiality of any comic are "inescapably, a metaphor for the subjectivity of perception" (21).

As well as using colour metaphorically, Dillon also makes stylistic choices that allow the reader to see Nao's perspective. The images and words on the page vividly evoke Nao's point of view and obsessive thoughts, which simultaneously negate her worth as an individual and her desire to be approved by her mother (Figure 5.2). At one point, close-up images of Nao's mother (who does not feature elsewhere in the memoir except in Nao's obsessive thoughts) are interspersed with short text boxes that reiterate Nao's self-deprecating thoughts and reassuring statements such as "Mum loves me" (Dillon 14). Here, in the first panel specifically, Dillon angles the image in a way that the reader observes the mother through Nao's eyes. The visual synecdoche deployed in the second panel, where the protagonist's face is only partially represented, clarifies the context of the protagonist's childhood. The random placement of the text boxes, over the image and even across the gutter space, also serves a temporal function as the image forces the reader to envision a younger Nao's perspective while the words strewn across the page represent her present thoughts.

This stylistic choice represents the complexities of Nao's struggle with OCD, which is characterised by perceptions of temporal shifts from past to present and vice versa. As Toombs argues that the immediate experience of the patient "occurs in inner time and, as such, it is not measurable according to the units of objective time scale" (232), so this stylistic metaphor represents the embodied experience of an OCD patient who experiences 'memory mixing' due to "altered dopaminergic activity in the cortico-striatal circuits involved in timing and time perception" (Gu and Kukreja 2). Several studies have suggested that since OCD patients are generally 'less confident' in their memories and lack 'memory vividness,' rituals and repetitive actions are developed as coping mechanisms to enrich a memory episode (Moritz and Jaeger 291, 296). In this case, the short phrases such as "Mum loves me" that are strewn across the page and reappear elsewhere in the memoir during a similar situation of extreme anxiety serve as indicators of Nao's ritualistic preoccupation with specific memories of her mother. Thus, the stylistic techniques that Dillon deploys—such as zooming, coupled with the scattering of phrases over the image—metaphorically map Nao's mental landscape during episodes of obsessive compulsions.

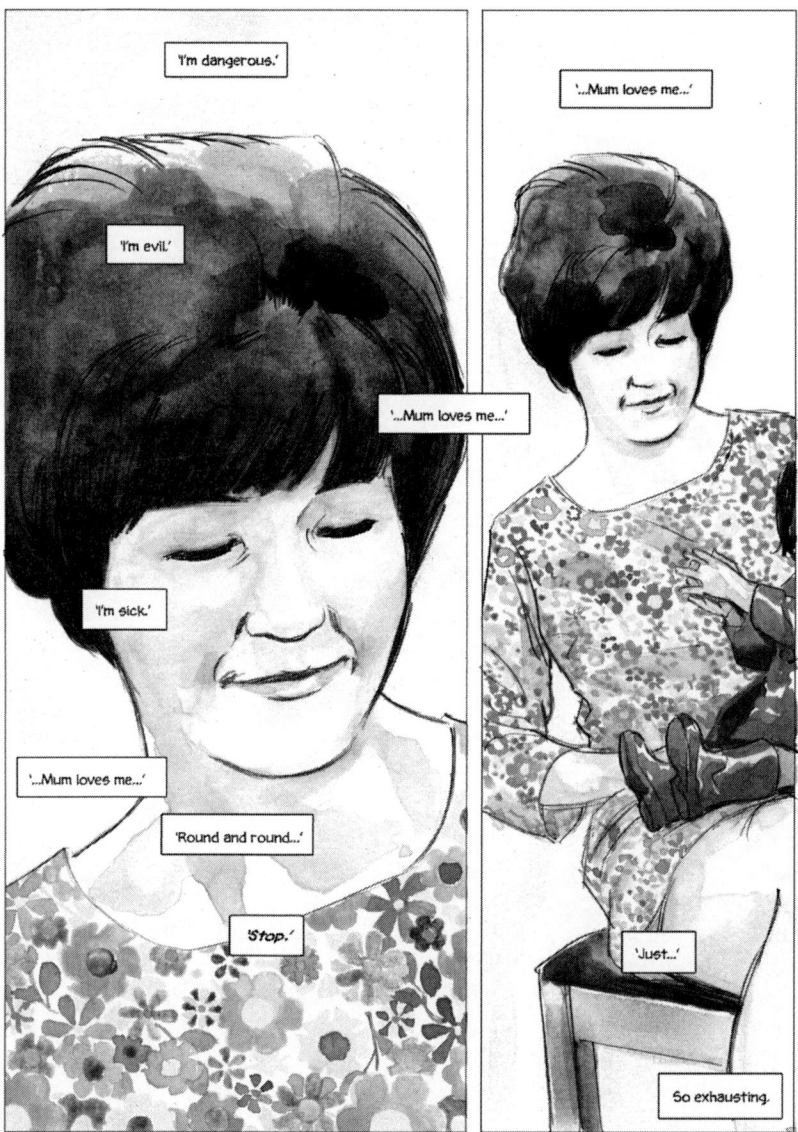

*Figure 5.2* Nao's obsessive thoughts on her mother (*The Nao of Brown*, p. 14).

## Traversing the Middle Ground through Visual Metaphors

In the context of mental disorders like schizophrenia, where patients' sense of the boundary between reality and hallucination is blurred, it is difficult to regard metaphors as a bridge between the subjective experiences of patients and the real world, but Kitayama argues that some people with schizophrenia are capable of creating new metaphors that enable them to communicate their experiences despite not necessarily sharing the same sense of reality as others (499). Unlike the available clinical descriptions of OCD and schizophrenia, which characterise patients' thoughts as "excessive" and "unreasonable" (Hudak and Dougherty 1) or even lacking emotion (Arozal et al. 57), Powell and Dillon reconfigure the patients' worlds in imaginative and emancipatory ways using spatial metaphors that mimic the fluidity of their mental landscapes. These graphic novels depart from the conventional narrative patterns of triumphalism/recovery or loss/death, instead traversing the middle ground between illness and health in a way that is informed by their authors' distinctive cultural identities. Nao negotiates her identity as a *hafu* living in Britain, whereas Ruth and Perry struggle to differentiate between external events and delusions that are related to the myths and superstitions that influenced Powell during his childhood in Arkansas, Mississippi, and Alabama (Elisabeth). Both Dillon and Powell shy away from closure in their narratives, instead celebrate a suggestive open-endedness. Both authors deploy metaphors to explore the middle ground of their protagonists' illness experience.

For instance, Powell deploys creative metaphors that are mapped directly to bodily experience. He elaborately illustrates Ruth's internal organs while she is lost in her thoughts during an interaction with Perry's friends (Figure 5.3). Although the boys are oblivious to Ruth's changing demeanour, the readers are exposed to her thoughts, which are depicted visually on the page. As Ruth is attracted to one of the boys in the gang, she feels that her love is "treasonous to [her delusional] insect suitors" which have become an inextricable part of her life world. Her thoughts about the insects' "backs, a softer abdomen, [and] shelled thorax" are mapped into her own bodily organs—a literal metamorphosis which actualises Ruth's imagination. Ruth's gestures and bodily posture convey a sense of lightness: she is shown with her hands loosely held like the limbs of an insect, her eyes closed, and her head drooping down. The image serves as a visual metaphor for the nature of the schizophrenic mind, which intermingles inner and outer reality.

In their article "Self-Disturbance in Schizophrenia," de Vries et al. argue that patients with schizophrenia experience "a disruption of the normal self-perception" where "tacit experiences intrude into the forefront of their attention, and the sense that inner-world experiences

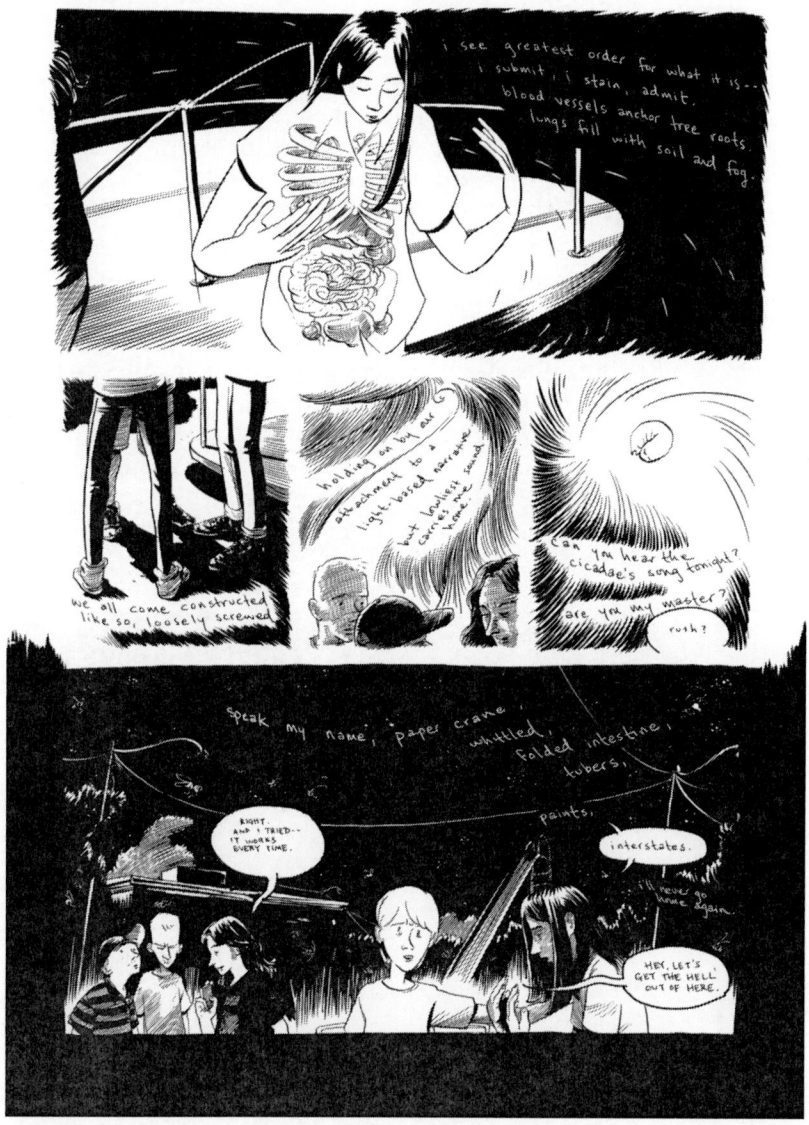

*Figure 5.3* Interspersing of inner and outer reality (*Swallow Me Whole*).

are private diminishes." Ruth experiences a similar intermingling of outer and inner worlds, which is delineated through her external bodily features and the floating text in the background that visually capture the feeble, rhythmic nature of her inner thoughts. Through such stylistic techniques, Powell creates a verbo-visual metaphor that approximately captures the experience of schizophrenia, which is then visually mapped onto Ruth's body and her surroundings.

Elsewhere, Powell experiments with the formal attributes of the medium of comics by introducing an indissoluble connection between the step-siblings Ruth and Perry. The shared nature of their hallucinations is visually manifested in sparse dialogue and captions (Figure 5.4). The two adjacent panels depict Perry and Ruth as children, encountering their delusionary creatures for the first time. The left panel shows Perry engaged in drawing and encountering the "little wizard" which he hallucinates to be what controls and dictates his actions, and the right panel shows Ruth's encounter with the cicada which begins to intrude into her thoughts. The characters in each panel are carefully aligned (Perry towards the left and Ruth towards the right) to suggest that one could not be fully characterised without the other. This arrangement illustrates what El Refaie refers to as "compositional spatial metaphor" (103) where panels, images, and words are arranged in a particular order to evoke metaphorical meanings.

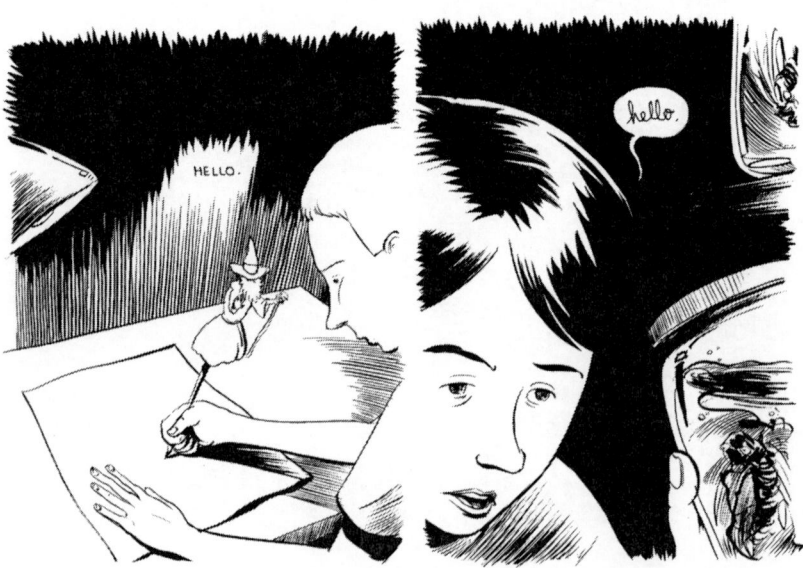

*Figure 5.4* Perry and Ruth in a single layout (*Swallow Me Whole*).

Here, Thierry Groensteen's principles of "arthrology" (linear relation of panels to each other) and "braiding" (connection across the multiframe of the page of a comic) help us to understand the metaphorical meanings that Powell intends to convey (Beaty and Nguyen). Although the linear relationship between the two panels invokes the siblings' initiation into their delusional worlds, the page as a whole looks like a single panel in which the siblings are merged together to make a whole individual, because of the disjunction between the jagged panel frames. The use of the merging of the panels as a visual metaphor for the close connection between Perry and Ruth suggests that they share a composite or conjoined identity. In essence, Powell uses a stylistic visual metaphor that connotes the shared subjective experience of the siblings during their childhood together. As Powell remarks in an interview with tfaw.comics, the siblings' shared subjective experience is 'magical' in that they seem more like "a sibling cult with its own mythology, language, ritual, and way of navigating the world" (Elisabeth).

Similarly, Dillon engages in a verbal and visual play on the word "brown" at the beginning of his narrative (Figure 5.5). Nao's childhood picture, which is pasted on the hallway of her mother's house, serves as a visual metaphor for the conflicts that she faced as a *hafu*. Dillon's deliberate choice of Justin Green's alter ego, Binky Brown, as a motif in this image also signifies Nao's future diagnosis of OCD. Although her friends regarded her as an "exotic other" (8), Nao is seen struggling to hide her illness, as we see from her clenched fists and hidden eyes. Dillon subtly suggests how "brown" defines Nao's identity as a *hafu* and her permanent inability to associate herself with black (evil) or white (good), which is a feature of her OCD. The page is replete with statements in text boxes that reveal how Nao struggled to negotiate these differing opinions about herself—she states that although she always accepted her boyfriends' comments on how "cute and cool [she] looks in the photo," she felt "torn" inside (8).

Although she seems like a "cute and quiet 'arty' type, half English, half Japanese," she exclaims that they are ignorant of the fact that she is "a fucking mental case" (8). These statements, which are strewn across the image, vividly convey her existence as a *hafu* diagnosed with OCD. The letter 'B,' which is etched on her t-shirt, not only suggests Nao's links with Binky Brown's predicament with regard to her illness; it also connotes her final realisation that "things aren't so black and white after all. In fact, they're much more ... brown" (Cover copy). Like Powell, Dillon resists every attempt to categorise his protagonist's experience into rigid categories of good and evil or black and white. Instead, here, the visual metaphor constructed through

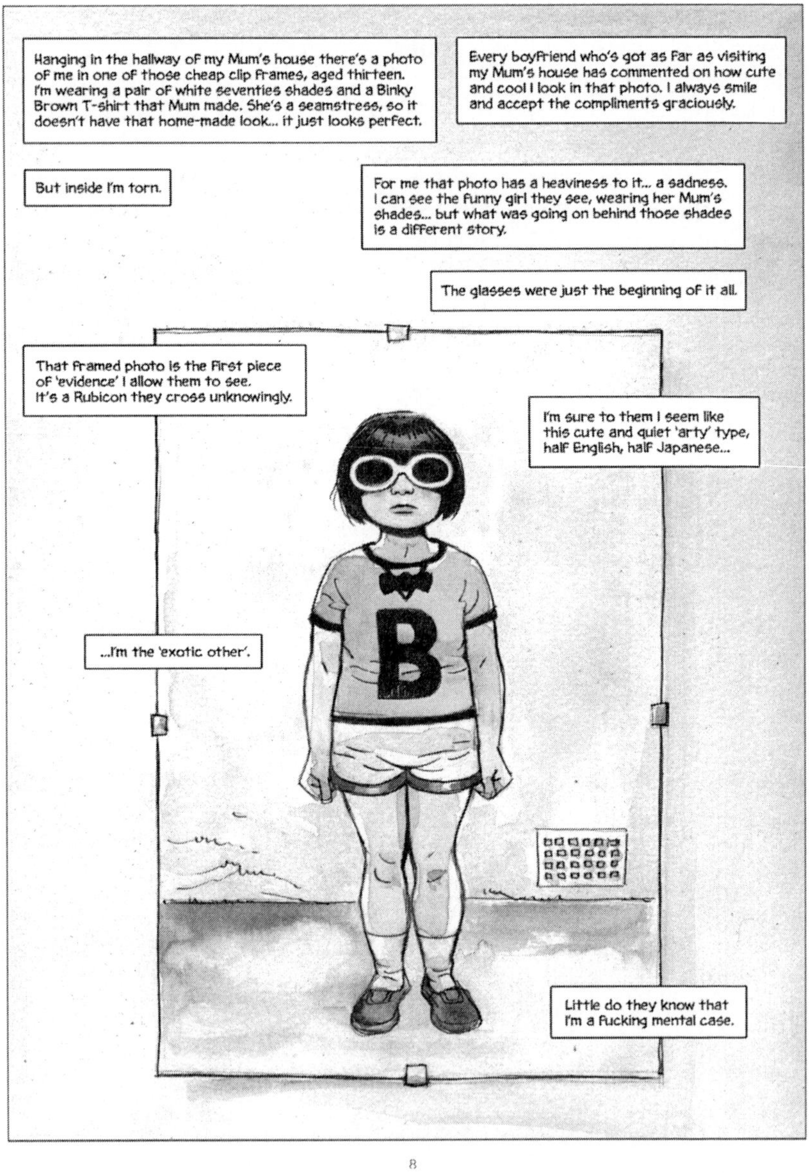

*Figure 5.5*  Nao's childhood image at her mother's house (*The Nao of Brown*, p. 8).

colour and literary allusions evokes the sense of in-betweenness which is characteristic of the protagonist's identity.

## Conclusion

In their graphic narratives, Powell and Dillon deftly transform their illness experience into creative and insightful journeys. Drawing inspiration from accounts of the real-life experiences of friends and relatives with schizophrenia and OCD, these authors have attempted to recreate the inner world of such people through stylistic and spatial visual metaphors. As well as bringing to life patients' subjective experiences, *Swallow Me Whole* and *The Nao of Brown* radically foreground marginal perspectives on illness, contrasting them with the plethora of scientific prescriptions and cultural prejudices that limit the life of sufferers.

The relationship between the sick and the healthy evolves into a productive and symmetrical encounter only when both parties realise the significance of their mutually imbricated identities. Such an awareness not only neutralises negative stereotypes about illness but also alleviates the patients' quandaries. The socio-cultural chasm between the healthy and sick in clinical contexts, where the sick are seen as inferior, can only be bridged by debate grounded in mutual respect for the diverse perspectives on health and illness. In other words, if patients, doctors, and caregivers were to eschew epistemic injustice by "suspend[ing] the belief in the reality of an objective disease entity," and "[s]hifting the focus … toward the [illness] experience" (Carel 200), they could access novel aspects of the experience of mental illness. Acknowledgement of the patient's essential role in defining an illness would lead professional and non-professional caregivers to regard patients as cognitively reliable, allowing them to spend ample time with patients in neutral yet intimate contexts.

Visual metaphors help to disentangle the intricate patterns of patients' mental landscapes which do not fit narratives of triumph or loss. These metaphors stylistically and spatially delineate the subjective experience of patients in viscerally engaging ways, thus capturing the particularities of the experience of mental illness. The metaphors in Dillon's narrative clarify Nao's struggle with her cultural identity as a *hafu* and her obsessions about good and evil, whereas Powell deploys visual metaphors which bring to life Ruth's and Perry's hallucinatory worlds and their impact on Ruth's and Perry's everyday life. By amalgamating patients' interpretations of the past and anticipations of the future, these graphic narratives represent the lived experience of illness within the framework of their characters' unique mental dispositions. In so doing, they move away from objectifying illness as 'disease' to "a reflective description" which is "transcendent to subjective consciousness" (Toombs 239).

## Acknowledgement

This chapter is derived in part from an article published in the *Journal of Graphic Novels and Comics* on 24 August 2020 © Taylor & Francis, available online: https://doi.org/10.1080/21504857.2020.1809482.

## Reference List

Angermeyer, Matthias C., and Herbert Matschinger. "The Stereotype of Schizophrenia and Its Impact on Discrimination Against People with Schizophrenia: Results From a Representative Survey in Germany." *Schizophrenia Bulletin*, vol. 30, no. 4, 2004, pp. 1049–1061.

Arozal, Wawaimuli, et al. "Treatment Patterns of Antipsychotics and Clinical Features for Treating Patients with Schizophrenia at the Teaching Hospital in Jakarta, Indonesia." *Journal of Applied Pharmaceutical Science*, vol. 9, no. 2, 2019, pp. 57–63.

Baer, Lee. *Getting Control: Overcoming Your Obsessions and Compulsions.* Plume, 2012.

Beaty, Bart, and Nick Nguyen, translators. *The System of Comics.* By Theirry Groensteen, UP of Mississippi, 2007.

Carel, Havi. *Phenemenology of Illness.* Oxford UP, 2016.

Charon, Rita. *Narrative Medicine: Honoring the Stories of Illness.* Oxford UP, 2006.

Cohn, Neil. "Being Explicit about the Implicit: Inference Generating Techniques in Visual Narrative." *Language and Cognition*, vol. 11, 2019, pp. 66–97.

Cover copy. *The Nao of Brown*, by Glyn Dillon, Self Made Hero, 2012.

de Vries, Rob de et al. "Self-Disturbance in Schizophrenia: A Phenomenological Approach to Better Understand Our Patients." *The Primary Care Companion for CNS Disorders*, vol. 15, no. 1, 2013. doi: 10.4088/PCC.12m01382.

Dillon, Glyn. *The Nao of Brown.* SelfMadeHero, 2012.

El Refaie, Elisabeth. *Visual Metaphor and Embodiment in Graphic Illness Narratives.* Oxford UP, 2019.

Elisabeth. "Nate Powell on Swallow Me Whole, Mental Illness & the Magic of Siblings." *Tfaw.comics*, 25 August 2010, https://blog.tfaw.com/2010/08/25/nate-powell-on-swallow-me-whole-mental-illness-the-magic-of-siblings/.

Fileva, Iskra. *Questions of Character.* Oxford UP, 2017.

Fineberg, Naomi A., and Dan J. Stein. *Obsessive Compulsive Disorder.* Oxford UP, 2007.

Gu, Bon-Mi, and K. Kukreja. "Obsessive-Compulsive Disorder and Memory-Mixing in Temporal Comparison: Is Implicit Learning the Missing Link?" *Frontiers in Integrative Neuroscience*, no. 5, 2011. *PubMed.* doi: 10.3389/fnint.2011.00038.

Hudak, Robert, and Darin D. Dougherty, editors. *Clinical Obsessive-Compulsive Disorders in Adults and Children.* Cambridge UP, 2011.

Kitayama, Osamu. "Metaphorization—Making Terms." *The International Journal of Psychoanalysis*, vol. 68, no. 4, 1987, pp. 499–509.

Li, Jie, et al. "Stigma and Discrimination Experienced by People with Schizophrenia Living in the Community in Guangzhou, China." *Psychiatry Research*, vol. 255, 2017, pp. 225–231.

Moritz, Steffen, and Anne Jaeger. "Decreased Memory Confidence in Obsessive–Compulsive Disorder for Scenarios High and Low on Responsibility: Is Low Still Too High?" *European Archives of Psychiatry and Clinical Neuroscience*, vol. 268, no. 3, 2017, pp. 291–299. doi: 10.1007/s00406-017-0783-0.

Parnas, Josef, and Mads Gram Henriksen. "Mysticism and Schizophrenia: A Phenomenological Exploration of the Structure of Consciousness in the Schizophrenia Spectrum Disorders." *Consciousness and Cognition*, vol. 43, 2016, pp. 75–88.

Postmes, Lot, et al. "Schizophrenia as a Self-Disorder due to Perceptual Incoherence." *Schizophrenia Research*, vol. 152, 2014, pp. 41–50.

Powell, Nate. *Swallow Me Whole.* TopShelf, 2008.

Tompkins, Michael A. *OCD: A Guide for the Newly Diagnosed.* New Harbinger, 2012.

Toombs, S. Kay. "The Temporality of Illness: Four Levels of Experience." *Theoretical Medicine*, vol. 11, 1990, pp. 227–241.

Troup, Christina. "Interview: Nate Powell on 'Swallow Me Whole'." *ComicMix*, 1 November 2008, https://www.comicmix.com/2008/11/01/interview-nate-powell-on-swallow-me-whole/.

Wolk, Douglas. *Reading Comics: How Graphic Novels Work and What They Mean.* Da Capo P, 2007.

Yılmaz, Emine, and A. Okanlı. "The Effect of Internalized Stigma on the Adherence to Treatment in Patients with Schizophrenia." *Archives of Psychiatric Nursing*, vol. 29, no. 5, 2015, pp. 297–301.

# 6  Visualising the Fragmented Selves
## Conventional and Creative Metaphors of Depression

## Introduction

Graphic memoirs on mental illness find expression through the unique semiotic nature of comics, which facilitates the encapsulation of complex psychicscapes and embodiment of the artist's experiences. In so doing, these verbo-visual techniques provide vividness, translating the sufferer's altered mental perspective effectively for the reader. The deployment of such elements inherent in the medium facilitates multi-layered connections to the patient's narrative which provide a depth beyond the raw medical discourse, and thereby reconfigures the extant perceptions surrounding mental illness. The creative metaphors that these authors use in their graphic memoirs reflect the multiple realities as experienced by the sufferer and are not restrained by the binary logic of recovery or continued suffering. As such, graphic memoirs like Allie Brosh's *Hyperbole and a Half: Unfortunate Situations, Flawed Coping Mechanisms, Mayhem, and other Things That Happened* (2013; hereafter, *Hyperbole*), Darryl Cunnigham's *Psychiatric Tales: Eleven Graphic Stories About Mental Illness* (2011; hereafter, *Psychiatric Tales*), and Brick's *Depresso: Or: How I Learned to Stop Worrying and Embrace Being Bonkers* (2010; hereafter, *Depresso*), which describe their personal experiences of living with depression, make a profound investment in the unique attributes of comics through the use of pictorial and stylistic metaphors. The present chapter, with reference to the abovementioned graphic memoirs on depression, investigates the mediative value of conventional and creative rhetorical devices which are unique to the medium of comics. Drawing on theoretical insights from Lakoff and Johnson and other graphic theorists like Williams and El Refaie, this chapter scrutinises how these metaphors aid the memoirists in actualising the subjective experience of their mental illness.

DOI: 10.4324/9781003214229-7

Brosh's *Hyperbole* in 19 chapters traces the various stages of the author's depression in a purposefully crude art style. Brosh's memoir originally was serialised in her blog which received immense reception and appreciation for the portrayal of depression. Cunningham, on the other hand, in *Psychiatric Tales* chronicles a range of experiences as a healthcare worker in a psychiatric ward. The stark black and white drawings and visual metaphors that delineate 11 episodes drawn from his experiences engage the reader in urgent and visceral ways. This chapter specifically focusses on a chapter titled, "Depression," which delineates Cunningham's own struggle with depression. Brick a.k.a. Tom Freeman's *Depresso* documents the depressive phase of his life in literal and metaphorical ways which creatively foreground multiple realities that depressed individuals encounter. The vital blend of verbal and visual modes in the comic medium grants these artists myriad ways of representing the human mind altered by mental illness. Distancing themselves from the cliched notions of mental illness as untranslatable and not amenable for representation, these graphic memoirs actualise the nuances of their respective authors' experiences, through both conventional and creative tropes.

Several other graphic narratives of mental illness, such as Clem Martini's *Bitter Medicine: A Graphic Memoir of Mental Illness* (2010), Steven Struble's *Li'l Depressed Boy* (2011), and Elaine Will's *Look Straight Ahead* (2013), exploit imagery as well as visual rhetorical devices (such as metaphors) to define and effectively relate their mental states. Attesting to the complex relationship between "the sequence of events happening (chronology) and the sequence in which they are narrated (narrative line)," Bredehoft argues that comics offer the possibility of a narrative mode that disrupts the uni-directional and irreversible chronology of other media. The two-dimensional architecture of a comic page "allows comics narration to break the linearity of a time-sequenced narrative line" (872). In fact, comics allow the author to recount experiences in narrative/subjective time sequence against the ideal of chronological/objective time, providing a more faithful rendition. Drawing from distinct artistic genres and traditions, comic artists have often exploited a wide range of spatio-temporal frames and rhetorical devices in order to effectively translate their perceptions. In particular, graphic artists have resorted to visual strategies such as layout and panelling that are unavailable in exclusively verbal narratives, in order to depict the intricacies and abstract ambits of the mental illness experience in metaphorical ways.

## Conventional and Creative Metaphors of Depression

The metaphors in many of the graphic memoirs are developed through two dominant ways, utilising conventional patterns from the available image bank and generating new metaphors essential for conveying the singular experience of the illness. The 'image bank of metaphors' refers to conventional metaphors already available to the comic artist in depicting illness. For instance, commonly used metaphors for depression include a body pressed down by weight, falling, crashing, or being entrapped in a three-dimensional space, such as a pit, hole, or bubble (El Refaie, "Looking" 154). Frank Gilliam and others in *Depression and Brain Dysfunction* use the etymological link of the term 'depression' to the Latin *deprimere*, meaning 'to press down,' to underscore its "metaphorical origin" (5). On the basis of their subjective peculiarities and experiences, artists either modify/redraw existing metaphors or generate new ones that more succinctly encapsulate perspectives on their illness. In devising distinct and novel metaphors, graphic memoirists convey a complex corporeal and affective experience of their specific illness. For instance, Brian Fies' graphic memoir, *Mom's*

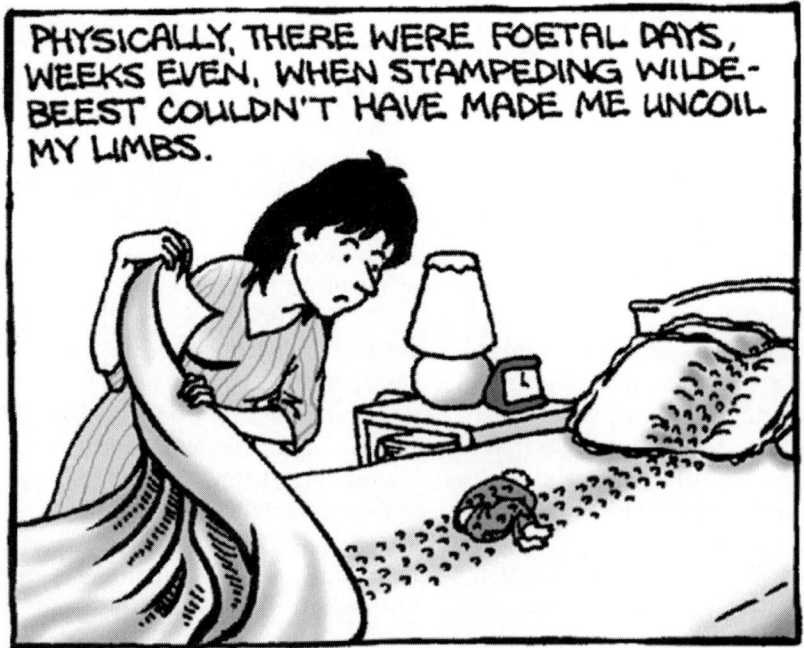

*Figure 6.1* Tom's "foetal days" (*Depresso*, p. 86).

*Cancer*, about his mother's lung cancer, uses several visual game metaphors in order to convey the uncertainty of the cancer experience and also to highlight "the teetering on the edge state of mind and near-to-death experience of his mother" (Venkatesan and Peter). Fies projects his mother's mental state during chemotherapy as that of a funambulist with a vulture and an elephant on either ends of a balancing pole. Such a metaphor allows Fies to clarify the uncertainties of chemotherapy and treatment in text boxes, with the visuals metaphorically equating his mother's cancer experience to that of a "balancing act" (Fies 60).

Brick delineates his experience with mental illness through metaphors drawn from the existing image bank of depression. Drawing from the iconography of depression characterised by "slumped shoulders" and "expressionless face" (Czerwiec et al. 125), Brick represents himself lying in a foetal position on a couch (Figure 6.1) to convey passivity and introversion caused by depression. His immobile corpse-like figure connotes the impact of depression which constrains him both physically and mentally. At the height of his depressive mental state, Brick "shrink[s] to minute proportions [and lies] in a fetal position in bed" (Williams 79).

In a similar manner, borrowing from the existing image bank of the slump body posture, Brosh's avatar reclines on a sofa with negligible change in posture in subsequent panels. In fact, the repeated use of the same avatar with staring eyes and the curved down lips denote "the long-lasting metaphor … of the mind, head, or body pressed or weighed down by a burden" (El Refaie, "Looking" 154). Although both Brick and Brosh use the slouched body as a metaphor for depression, they invoke them in different ways. Accordingly, while Brick's lack of facial expressions suggests the void and his inability to move, the depiction of Brosh's avatar in almost identical panels arranged in two distinct columns signifies her fragmented identity. In the right-hand section of the panels, Brosh is seen as lethargic and worried. She is constantly being berated and accused by her 'normal' healthy self. It can be assumed that Brosh has internalised the patronising influence of society which dismisses any delegitimised behaviour. As such, Brosh is constantly threatened by her alter ego who commands her to "stop being sad" (Brosh, *Hyperbole* 101). Moreover, the fact that both figures are turned towards one direction, and not towards each other, creates a sense of temporal stasis, implying that Brosh's efforts to talk herself out of depression are not fruitful (El Refaie, *Visual Metaphor* 176). The dichotomy created between the depressed and the 'normal' self is amplified in the illustration. Not only does such a representation draw attention to the different realities that are external to

Brosh's experience of depression, but it also embodies her fragmented/ split self. Such repetitive panel/frame arrangement acts as a compositional spatial metaphor which integrates the conceptual metaphor DEPRESSION IS DOWN/FRAGMENTED.

Demonstrating Whitlock's contention that visual images "relay affect and invoke a moral and ethical responsiveness in the viewer regarding the suffering of others" (965), Brosh's avatar not only conveys the author's depressed mental state but also allows a community of sufferers of depression to relate to her experience. Establishing a relationship between the cartoon art style and the reader in terms of identification and universality, McCloud in his book *Understanding Comics* states that: "the more cartoony a face is … the more people it could be said to describe" (31). Most of the comments that Brosh received in response to her webcomics since their inception reflect readers' easy identification with Brosh's embodied self, illustrated as a cartoon.[1] In an interview with *Goodreads*, Brosh clarifies her choice of cartoon imagery thus, "it's important that it doesn't look realistic" (Brosh, "Interview"). Thus, the staring blank eyes and the thin line appendages of Brosh's avatar communicate a 'lack of feeling' (Brosh, *Hyperbole* 124), which is characteristic of depression. Brosh's unique art style and humour has been lauded by Chute in her recent work *Why Comics: From Underground to Everywhere*, stating that "Brosh is prodigiously talented, as her unique humor and aesthetic make evident—and she without question touched a nerve, and galvanized a community, by so directly addressing depression through comics" (264). Chute further comments on the expressivity that Brosh's simple art style achieves in representing her depressed condition, affirming that "Brosh taps into cartooning's signature power: distilling and condensing essence through line" (268). Though minimalist in style, Brosh's drawings reflect her internal reality succinctly by capturing a concept that is otherwise too abstract to articulate.

Another conventional mode of conceptualising depressed self as fractured/split is found in Brick's *Depresso*. In the chapter titled "Enter the Dragon," Brick's comic avatar Tom encounters a giant lizard which he refers to as a "mutant gecko" and a "guardian angel" (40). Although the lizard appears to be a distinct fictional character in the memoir, it is always pictured alongside Tom (Figure 6.2). Moreover, the conversations between the lizard and Tom is mostly introspective and Tom addresses the lizard by his own name (64). Thus, the lizard metaphorically represents Tom's externalised depressed self which he considers distinct from his healthy self. As evident from the figure, the pain that Tom experiences during reflexology impacts the giant lizard in a greater degree. In the second tier, the lizard even

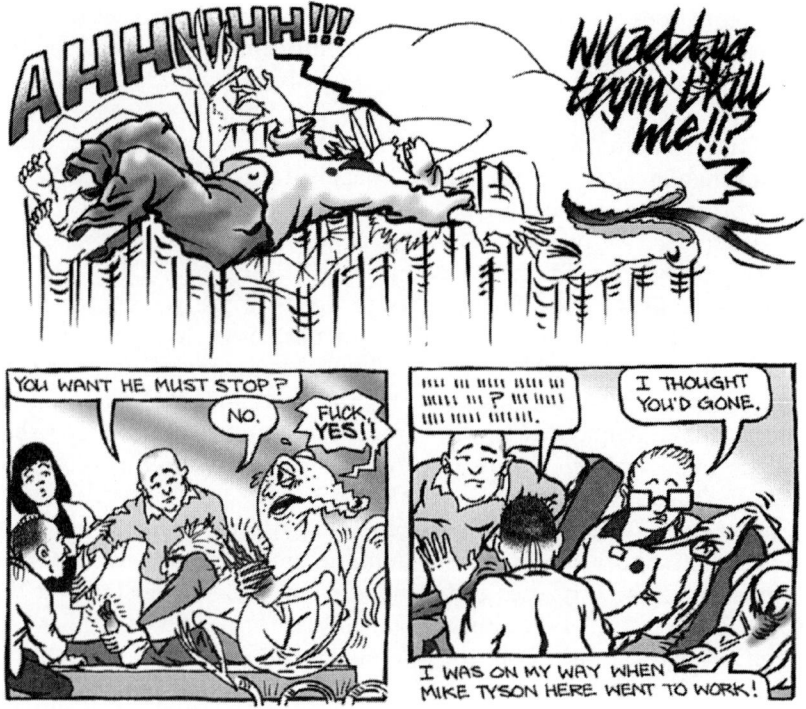

*Figure 6.2* Tom at the massage center (*Depresso*, p. 70).

disagrees with Tom who wants to be cured of his illness condition although both are pictured alongside each other with similar gestures that suggest pain. Thus, Tom's depressed/fragmented self appears to be part of and different from Tom at the same time. Drawing from the metaphorical connotations to lizards as omens of disaster (Hurwit 128), Brick pictures his depressed and fragmented mental state as a fire-breathing dragon that evokes the torturous phases of the illness condition (Brick 101).

As Matthew Ratcliffe and Achim Stephan observe in *Depression, Emotion and the Self: Philosophical and Interdisciplinary Perspectives*, depression causes patients to experience themselves as "blurred and fragmented, which provokes excruciating feelings of incoherence, emptiness, uncertainty, and inauthenticity" (158). Tom undergoes similar phases of fragmented sense of identity throughout the memoir as he is compelled to negotiate even mundane routines with the giant lizard a.k.a his alter ego which is overly scrupulous and critical of everything that Tom does. The visual metaphor of the lizard/dragon thus signifies the negative and distressing aspects of depression by drawing from the conventional allusions to myths and symbols (Hurwit 123).

Similarly, Cunningham's *Psychiatric Tales* portrays several visual metaphors that suggest the fragility of his mind during depression. Cunningham struggles to maintain his mental balance when he starts to work as a mental health nurse while attempting to comprehend his own depressive symptoms. The fragility that Cunningham experiences during such instances of intense pressure is traced to objects that are illustrated as broken. His inability to hold himself together is illustrated via a visual metaphor of a broken glass sheet that is at the brink of falling into pieces. The subsequent tier shows a pencil that is broken into two pieces with a caption—"my life as a nurse was over and I'd been unable to make anything of myself as an illustrator" (133)—that suggests the apprehensions regarding his career as an illustrator and the destructive ways in which his illness impacts his creativity (El Refaie, *Visual Metaphor* 175). Such recurrent patterns of fragility in these visual metaphors contextualise Cunningham's mental condition. The captions to these images of fragile and fragmented objects and the clear background of the panels in which these are depicted further distinguish these scenes from the plotline and contextualise the author's depressed mental state. Such conventional metaphors of depression are commonly used by sufferers of depression. For instance, a study by Fullagar and O'Brien reveals that sufferers of depression in Australia often describe their mental state thus: "falling, going downhill, crashing, or descending into a state of depression" (1066). Brick also deploys the conceptualisation of depression as breaking apart/falling. In Figure 6.3, Tom is illustrated as an astronaut inside a space ship which breaks apart due to mounting pressure. Metaphorically, Brick clarifies in the caption that the space ship refers to his life which once was "ordered and arranged" (87). At the level of form, Brick elucidates his mental condition by framing the panels depicting the metaphor in jagged lines as opposed to the neat boxes which portray the actual events. The enormity of the mental break-down is further accentuated in the central tier which depicts the crashing space ship without a panel frame.

In the absence of conventional relations of concepts, artists often yoke two distinct notions for conveying subtle subjective emotions. In particular, the illustration of unique mentalscapes and perspectives necessitates the creation of novel metaphors that can adequately encapsulate the intricacies of the author's experience. These creative metaphors are neither restricted to triumphalism nor failure patterns

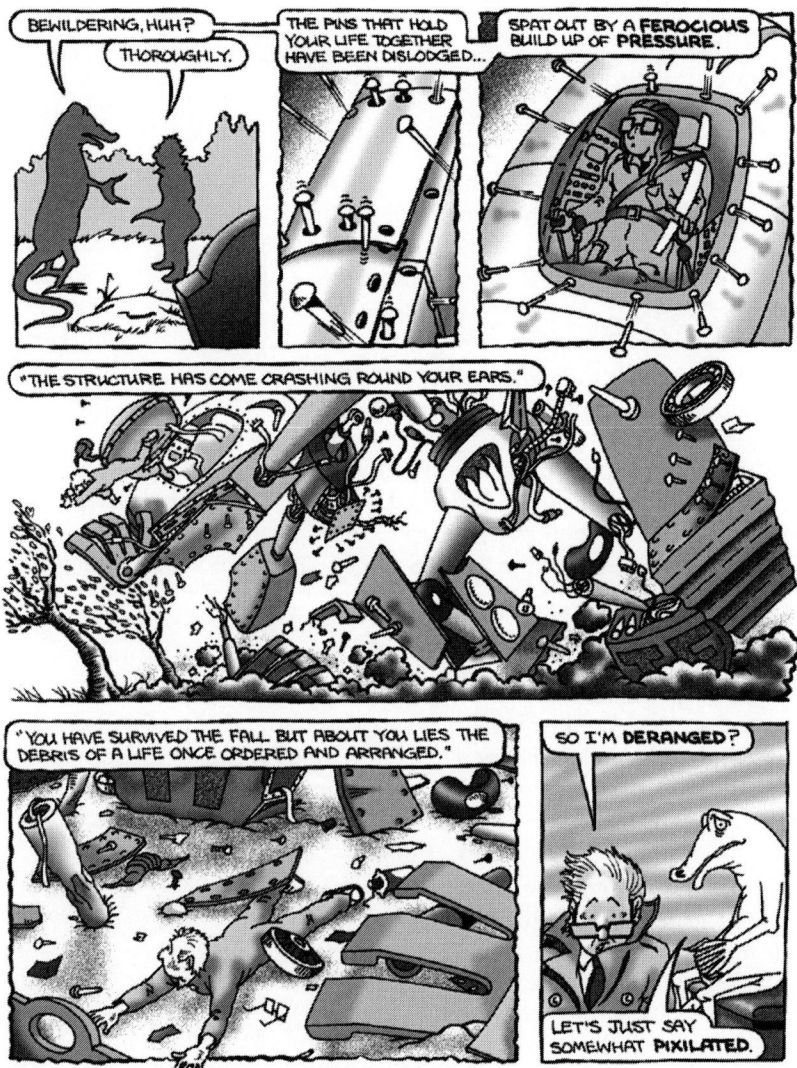

*Figure 6.3* Tom's depressive episode (*Depresso*, p. 87).

but purely convey the stark reality of surviving in the middle ground between life and death. As Thembeck remarks,

[t]hese new metaphors of illness thus neither lead to the excessive beatification nor to the condemnation of sick subjects. Instead,

they simply reflect the reality that no matter how evolved our medical practices, disease and death remain present as facts that need to be acknowledged and eventually negotiated in the process of living.

(277–278)

For instance, distinct from the biomedical repertoire of illustrations for depression which focus on the patient's slouched posture and drooped down facial features (Ogle e3), Cunningham uses several pictorial and stylistic metaphors to delineate the depressive phases of his illness.

Cunningham illustrates his mood states with sparse facial features and by experimenting with black and white shades. In the depressed state, his images perform a modifying function where his isolation is foregrounded by the stark contrasts of black and white patterns. The images not only diagram Cunningham's depressive symptoms, which are distinct from the ordained verbal/visual symbols of depression (with the slumped body posture and face resting on palm of the hand), but also economically summarise the nuances of his subjective experience of the illness. For instance, the social anxiety, tension, and fear that Cunningham experiences during depression are signified using zig-zag lines in the background and the striped pattern on his shirt which simulates prison bars which restrict him from maintaining social relationships. In essence, such an attempt starkly distinguishes Cunningham's personal narration from the symptomatic and apathetic prescriptions of biomedicine. In addition, these stylistic metaphors capture the intricacies of the depressed psychic state and establishes multi-layered connections to the narrative.

Brosh's creative metaphors make her mental illness discernible in simple line drawings. One of the popular episodes in *Hyperbole* is her negotiation with a group of people who intend to save her from depression. The entire exercise turns futile as Brosh is struggling to explain her depression while others are already in the process of suggesting ways to fix it in their own terms. In the meantime, Brosh has lost access to her emotions as she exclaims, "I feel nothing" (Brosh, *Hyperbole* 124). To relate her struggle with depression and her futile attempts to communicate the condition with others, Brosh uses the verbo-visual metaphor of a dead fish. As El Refaie contends, in verbo-visual metaphors, "pictures are completely reliant on verbal text for their metaphorical potential" (*Visual Metaphor* 99). In speech balloons, Brosh compares her experience to "having a bunch of dead fish, but no one around you will acknowledge that the fish are dead" (Brosh, *Hyperbole* 132). In spite of Brosh's attempts to convince others of her helplessness with depression, each one provides their solution, such as feeding the dead fish to making them live again. The metaphor captures the illogicality and futility of such responses. Accentuating the impact of her helplessness, Brosh subsequently portrays herself as cornered in a blank background talking to her 'dead fish,' "it's ok fish ... it's gonna be okay" (Brosh, *Hyperbole* 136). The emptiness that Brosh experiences within is literally mapped into the space of the page, which is in stark contrast to the previous crowded panel. The metaphor of the dead fish conveys the legitimacy of a depressed individual's struggle, which is often considered invalid and rendered meaningless by others.

## Stylistic Metaphors of Depression

Graphic memoirists communicate the affective facets of the human mind through a variety of visual elements unique to comics. While both image and words contribute in the comic medium, it is the creative use of comics' formal elements or "pictorial runes" (Forceville and Eduardo 245) such as emanatas, special effects lettering, motion lines, and distinct panel shapes that enhance the content. In particular, these techniques that elaborate on the meanings encoded in multiple semiotic systems within the medium also function as stylistic metaphors. Emanatas have been used extensively as auxiliary descriptors that make characters and inanimate figures more expressive for underground comix artists of the 1960s. Notably, Robert Crumb and Aline Kominsky-Crumb captured the "texture of lived life" (Chute, *Graphic Women* 35) using "non-mimetic, non-signifying, non-concrete, and non-specific" (Davies 9) signs to mark material and behavioural processes in comics. Explaining the function of emanatas in relaying mental states, Davies stated that emanatas are a "set of abstract symbology emerging from, usually, the head, the sensing part of the body, to indicate mental processes" (9).

Brick in *Depresso* uses an array of expressive non-diegetic graphic signs to relay his depressed condition, characterised by fear and bewilderment. As these signs drawn from the 'visual vocabulary of comics' are related to 'emotional/cognitive states,' according to Neil Cohn et al., they involve "metaphorical understanding due to their proximity to the head and face" (2). Semantically, the emanatas that often surround the head of Brick's comic avatar depict his emotions while the jagged speech balloons signify his exaggerated speech. Most of the frightening interludes that Tom experiences are rendered through emanatas, swirls, motion lines, and onomatopoeia, suggesting acute activity and confused state of his mind. For instance, the panels on the page rearrange themselves into varying sizes, inundated with plewds

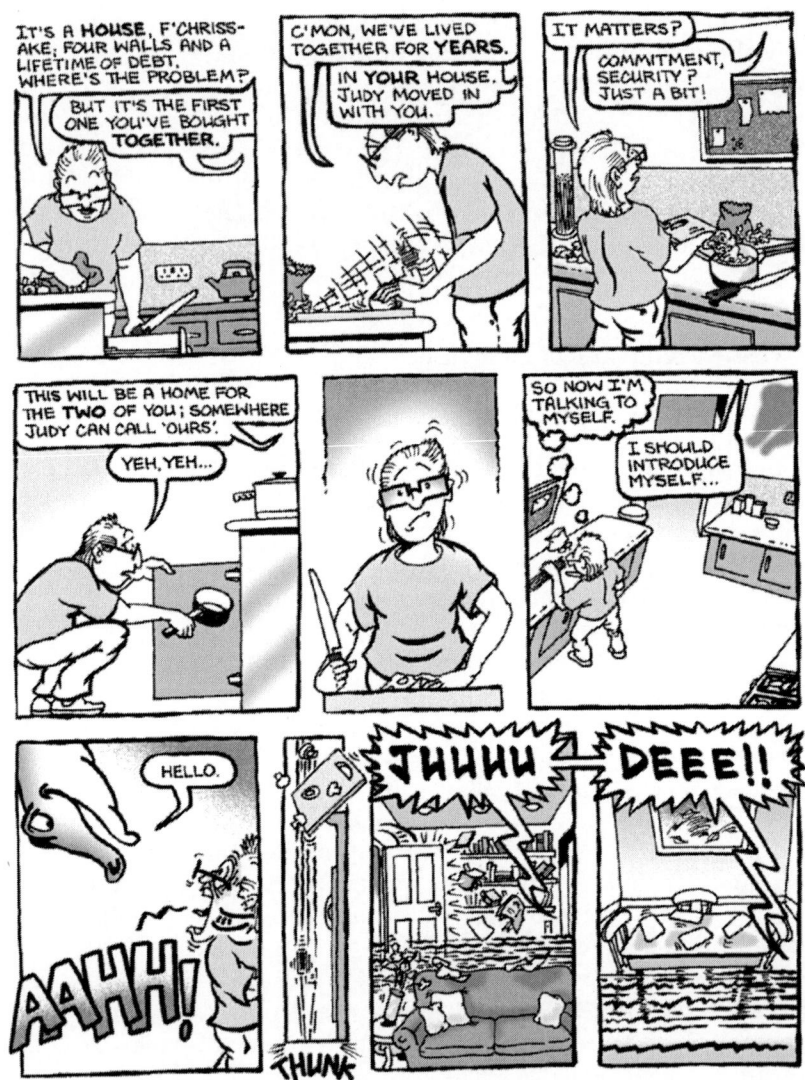

*Figure 6.4* Tom's first encounter with the giant lizard (*Depresso*, p. 35).

and motion lines to signify uncontrollable dread when Tom meets the giant lizard for the first time (Figure 6.4). Specifically, as Tom rushes out of the room screaming for help, the objects in the background fly out of the panel and the speech balloons that are framed with jagged tails resembling thunder strokes transgress the panel borders. Therefore, depiction of Tom's altered perspective towards the world around him is deeply reliant on the visual language of comics that convey his different embodied states. As McCloud argues, the idea that a picture/ sign can "evoke an emotional or sensual response in the viewer is vital to the art of comics" (121), and thus, they are "more a visual metaphor" than a picture or line (128).

Graphic artists also experiment with the structure and page layout to accentuate the meanings in the text. In the context of mental illness, the panel/page layout is generally rearranged into a chaotic structure to enhance the depiction of the incoherent and fluid mental states. For instance, artists across time have rejected definite latticed panel borders and embraced novel panel structures or panels without borders to portray psychic sequences in order to distinguish them from mundane/ objective episodes. For example, Craig Thompson's *Carnet de Voyage* (2004) experimented with panels without borders in order to depict instances of shock or extreme emotions. Forgoing generic boundaries, Thompson's sketchbook/travel diary represents his dissociative and fragmented mind by the use of chaotic and fluid page layouts. Thompson also utilises the comic live area to depict his emotional state and also to signify "immediacy, starkness, [and] directness" (Davies 11). Notably, while Thompson's exuberant mental activity is represented by unenclosed space on the page, the layout realigns to the grid format once his emotions are calmed and controlled.

Similarly, Brick experimented with the basic layout of comics so as to represent and formally align with his psychic response to varying mood states. As such, Brick orchestrates an interplay between the two distinct styles of comic page layout. On the one hand, diverse verbo-visual elements breaking free from the prescribed boundaries of the latticed structure and floating across the page align with Brick's mental state whenever he listens to music (Brick 98). The panels assume a musical quality as they float across the page along with musical notes and lyrics. By contrast, during treatment and counselling sessions, the page conforms to the traditional arrangement of panels (3 × 3 or 4 × 4 latticed panel arrangement) suggesting Brick's controlled psychic condition. Elsewhere, Brick deploys zoomed out splash pages with minimal details in the background to suggest disinterest and passivity that characterise depression. For instance, after a disappointing counselling episode, the subsequent splash page is creatively modulated, featuring Tom who is forced to fill numerous response sheets before leaving the counselling centre. Here, Brick's avatar is contained in a minimal space in the centre of the page surrounded by a fading cloud while the rest of the page is left blank. In deploying such stylistic techniques with limited use of emanatas, the page conveys notions of objectivity and precision that characterise clinical settings. The convergence of stylistic and semantic features in the comic grid illustrates Tom's vulnerable position during clinical encounters. Similar to Thompson's experiment on the page, Brick's adept deployment of the rhetorical mise-en-page allows the author to recreate his psychic landscape in both content and form.

## Conclusion

Official visual rhetoric (available in medical illustrations and X-rays) generates standardised models of illness. By contrast, graphic pathographies develop an alternative/counter visual narrative through its engagement with illness conditions. The cultural power of *Depresso*, *Psychiatric Tales*, and *Hyperbole* lies in the way they delineate the personal experiences of Brick, Cunningham, and Brosh in both content and form, as opposed to the biomedical approach that seeks to pathologise individuals. As pathographers, they share nuances and perspectives on clinical interventions through an idiosyncratic iconographic language constituted through diverse elements of the medium, such as visual imagery, metaphors, and self-portraiture. As McMullin observes, "representing [one's] body on the page on [one's] own terms is speaking truth to power," and, in doing so, they retrieve power over their body and symptomatology.

Brick's memoir admits the affected body into the narrative metaphorically as he represents himself as an individual with depression in distinct artistic styles. His self-portrait as a giant overbearing lizard, and abstract and cartoon-like during certain phases of depression are some of the ways through which Brick presents his identity against the official iconography of medical discourse. Through such wide-ranging artistic embodiment of the self, Brick deftly maps his abstract and private experiences into the comicscape. As Velentzas rightly observes, Brick's use of visual metaphors "manifests an attempt to visualize the sensation of mental illness." Similarly, Brosh in her deliberately crude art style 'speaks truth to power' as she unashamedly presents her inadequacies and failures which society dismisses as improper. In exploiting the immediate and resonant form of the medium, Brosh struggles openly against the prejudices surrounding depression. Cunningham, on the other hand, *owns* the diagnosis of depression through the creative stylistic metaphors that he deploys in the memoir as against the symptomatic verbal representations available in biomedical repertoires. In essence, as Squier remarks, comic embodiment "reveal[s] unvoiced relationships, unarticulated emotions, unspoken possibilities, and even unacknowledged alternative perspectives" ("Literature" 130).

As El Refaie observes, "the formal properties and sociocultural conventions of comics offer unique opportunities for sufferers of depression [or mental illness] to reinterpret conventional mappings in creative ways, thereby ... opening up the possibility of new meaning and understanding" ("Looking" 170). To conclude, the psychic states and affective realms of mental illness experience are encapsulated in *Depresso*, *Psychiatric Tales*, and *Hyperbole* through the efficacious choice of conventional and creative metaphors and other visual techniques that capture the full agony of depression. Borrowing from the existing image bank of metaphors, on the one hand, and generating modified or new ones, on the other, Brick, Cunningham, and Brosh translate their experiences into a visual engagement for the readers. Ultimately, these memoirs constitute an interface between the scope of images and words in depicting complex mentalscapes. In so doing, the authors not only grant a unique access to the tacit nature of their illness experience, but also viscerally and emotionally illustrate the labyrinthine realms of their psyche.

## Acknowledgement

Some portions of this chapter are previously published as a research article by Sage. See Venkatesan, Sathyaraj, and Sweetha Saji. "Drawing the mind: Aesthetics of representing mental illness in select graphic memoirs." *Health: An International Journal for Social Study of Health, Illness and Medicine*, vol. 25, no. 1, 2021, pp. 37–50. Copyright © The Authors 2019. DOI: 10.1177/1363459319846930.

## Notes

1 Over 5,000 comments that Brosh received to her blog post (*Hyperbole and a Half: Depression Part Two*: http://hyperboleandahalf.blogspot.in/2013/05/dep.ression-part-two.html) attests to the ease with which readers identified with her experience of depression. Here are two examples:

I relate to this far too much.
(Comment posted to hyperboleandahalf.blogspot.in
on 9 May 2013, Archana R.).

I have been in similar situations.
(Comment posted to hyperboleandahalf.
blogspot.in on 9 May 2013, EJ).

## Reference List

Bredehoft, Thomas A. "Comics Architecture, Multidimensionality, and Time: Chris Ware's Jimmy Corrigan: The Smartest Kid on Earth." *MFS Modern Fiction Studies*, vol. 52, no. 4, 2006, pp. 869–890.

Brick. *Depresso, Or, How I Learned to Stop Worrying and Embrace Being Bonkers!* Knockabout, 2010.

Brosh, Allie. *Hyperbole and a Half: Unfortunate Situations, Flawed Coping Mechanisms, Mayhem, and Other Things That Happened*. Simon & Schuster, 2013.

———. "Interview with Allie Brosh." *Goodreads*, 9 December 2013, http://www.goodreads.com/interviews/show/913.Allie_Brosh.

Chute, Hillary. *Graphic Women: Life Narrative and Contemporary Comics*. Columbia UP, 2010.

———. *Why Comics: From Underground to Everywhere*. Harper Collins, 2017.

Cohn, Neil, et al. "Meaning Above the Head: Combinatorial Constraints on the Visual Vocabulary of Comics." *Journal of Cognitive Psychology*, 2016, pp. 1–16. doi: 10.1080/20445911.2016.1179314.

Cunningham, Darryl. *Psychiatric Tales*. Blank Slate Books, 2010.

Czerwiec, M. K., et al. *Graphic Medicine Manifesto*. The Pennsylvania State UP, 2015.

Davies, Paul F. "Representing Experience in Comics: Carnet de Voyage." *Journal of Graphic Novels and Comics*, 2016, pp. 1–17. doi: 10.1080/21504857.2015.1131173.

El Refaie, Elisabeth. "Looking on the Dark and Bright Side: Creative Metaphors of Depression in Two Graphic Memoirs." *Auto/Biography Studies*, vol. 29, no. 1, 2014, pp. 149–174.

———. *Visual Metaphor and Embodiment in Graphic Illness Narratives*. Oxford UP, 2019.

Fies, Brian. *Mom's Cancer*. Abrams Comicarts, 2006.

Forceville, Charles, and Urios-Aparisi Eduardo, editors. *Multimodal Metaphor*. Mouton de Gruyter, 2009.

Fullagar, Simone, and Wendy O'Brien. "Immobility, Battles, and the Journey of Feeling Alive: Women's Metaphors of Self-Transformation through Depression and Recovery." *Qualitative Health Research*, vol. 22, no. 8, 2012, pp. 1063–1072.

Gilliam, Frank G., et al. *Depression and Brain Dysfunction*. Taylor & Francis, 2006.

Hurwit, Jeffrey M. "Lizards, Lions, and the Uncanny in Early Greek Art." Hesperia: *The Journal of the American School of Classical Studies at Athens*, vol. 75, no. 1, 2006, pp. 121–136.

McCloud, Scott. *Understanding Comics: The Invisible Art*. Harper Perennial, 1994.

McMullin, Sheila. "On Comics and Disability." *Word Gathering: A Journal of Disability Poetry and Literature*, vol. 9, no. 1, 2015. http://www.wordgathering.com/issue36/reading_loop/mcmullin.html.

Ogle, Zimbini, Liezl Koen, and Dana J. H. Niehaus. "The Development of the Visual Screening Tool for Anxiety Disorders and Depression: Addressing Barriers to Screening for Depression and Anxiety Disorders in Hypertension and/or Diabetes." *African Journal of Primary Health Care and Family Medicine*, vol. 10, no. 1, 2018, pp. e1–e6. doi: 10.4102/phcfm.v10i1.1721.

Ratcliffe, Matthew, and Achim Stephan, editors. *Depression, Emotion and the Self: Philosophical and Interdisciplinary Perspectives.* Imprint Academic, 2014.

Squier, Susan M. "Literature and Medicine, Future Tense: Making it Graphic." *Literature and Medicine,* vol. 27, no. 1, 2009, pp. 124–152.

Thembeck, Tamar. *Performative Autopathographies: Self-Representations of Physical Illness in Contemporary Art.* 2009. McGill U. PhD dissertation.

Toombs, S. Kay. "Illness and the Paradigm of Lived Body." *Theoretical Medicine*, vol. 9, 1988, pp. 201–226.

Velentzas, Irene. "Seeing the Sensation: Sketch-Journaling and the Embodiment of Mental Illness in Autographics." *ImageText*, vol. 9, no. 2, 2017. http://imagetext.english.ufl.edu/archives/v9_2/velentzas/.

Venkatesan, Sathyaraj, and Anu Mary Peter. "Life is a Game: Visual Metaphors in Brian Fies' Mom's Cancer." *Hekteon International: A Journal of Medical Humanities*, Fall. 2015, http://www.hektoeninternational.org/index.php?option=com_content&view=article&id=1983.

Whitlock, Gillian. "Autographics: The Seeing "I" of the Comics." *Mfs Modern Fiction Studies*, vol. 52, no. 4, 2006, pp. 965–979.

Williams, Ian. "Graphic Medicine: The Portrayal of Illness in Underground and Autobiographical Comics." *Medicine, Health and the Arts: Approaches to the Medical Humanities*, edited by Victoria Bates et al., Routledge, 2014, pp. 64–84.

# Conclusion

Graphic illness narratives on mental illness are replete with visual metaphors that effectively delineate the emotional distress of the mentally ill and the cultural factors that lead to their suffering. With increasing awareness on mental health and its related concerns on identity, depictions of the personal and social stigma of the mentally ill provide an invaluable framework for comprehending hierarchical, prejudicial, and depersonalising proclivities in medical and popular cultural discourses. A comprehensive understanding of marginal perspectives on mental illness through visual metaphors facilitates a deeper reading of graphic narratives beyond the broader categories of life writing or visual studies.

The present study has critically considered seven graphic narratives on mental illness. They include Nate Powell's *Swallow Me Whole* (2008), Brick's *Depresso* (2010), Darryl Cunnigham's *Psychiatric Tales* (2011), Ellen Forney's *Marbles* (2012), Glyn Dillon's *The Nao of Brown* (2012), Allie Brosh's *Hyperbole and a Half* (2013), and Rachel Lindsay's *Rx* (2018). These graphic narratives are analysed in three core chapters using McCloudian and Groensteenian close-reading models and the conceptual metaphor theory (CMT) proposed by Lakoff and Johnson. The intersection and implications of exclusionary patterns, reiteration of stereotyped representations of the mentally ill, the non-availability of subjective perspectives on mental illness in biomedical and popular representations, and the authors' resolutions that foreground their lived reality provide the critical frames. Besides the two fictional accounts, analysis of personal mental illness narratives articulates the major concerns that border on subjectivity, identity and sites of resistance within medical and popular cultural discourses.

Much of the critical studies on graphic narratives treat the patient vis-à-vis the question of pain and embodiment. Though such approaches are valid, very few studies have explored the representation

DOI: 10.4324/9781003214229-8

of mental illness in graphic memoirs through visual metaphors. Moreover, this study justifiably draws attention to the different kinds of visual metaphors present in these mental illness narratives that have been somewhat overlooked. By using Lakoff and Johnson's CMT, this study uncovers the broad spectrum of the mentally ills' experiences, a relatively undertheorised area in medical humanities. Furthermore, analysing conceptual metaphors in a non-verbal medium like comics becomes significant in validating CMT's claim that humans think in and live by metaphors rather than merely use them verbally.

The central concern of this book, therefore, is to theorise mental illness concerns from the patient's perspective via visual metaphors. The aim is to demonstrate that the mentally ill are often represented as either grotesquely exaggerated or overly romanticised across diverse media and biomedical discourses. Further, they have been disparaged as emotionally drained and unreasonable individuals, incapable of active social engagements, and against the healthy/sane society. In this context, this study aims to unsettle the sanity/insanity binary and its related patterns of fixed categories of normal/abnormal, which depersonalise the mentally ill. Finally, we consider the CMT as a productive approach towards these graphic narratives, because it not only enriches the metaphor theory, it also reveals patterns in comics that attribute affective and therapeutic meaning to the patient's lived experience.

With the preceding objectives, this study begins by cataloguing significant milestones in medical humanities and graphic medicine and analysing the appropriateness of contextualising the chosen graphic narratives on mental illness. The Introduction illustrates the limitations of extant studies on mental illness representations in dealing with unvoiced sociocultural and personal dimensions of living with the condition. Given the multiple ways in which popular and medical discourses intersect and shape the experiences of the mentally ill, it is demonstrated that such representations are prejudiced and exclusionary. In so doing, the chapter foregrounds the significance of patient-centric and experiential visual metaphors that are deployed in graphic memoirs by the mentally ill.

Chapter 1 introduces graphic medicine as an emerging interdisciplinary genre that productively engages health professionals and literary scholars in exploring diverse perspectives on illness and health. This chapter first traces the origins of the field in public-health-related cartoons from the eighteenth century, hagiographies of the 1940s, and confessional autobiographies like Green's *Binky Brown*, which definitively introduced narratives on illness. Next, the chapter establishes graphic medicine as an evolved genre of comics that vocalises marginal concerns on patient identity and healthcare practices. Yoking the tenets of comics and medicine, graphic medicine aims to promote patients', caregivers', and doctors' affective knowledge and subjective truths against the monolithic and reductive medical chart and text-based prescriptions. Therefore, the chapter proposes graphic medicine as an alternative body of medical knowledge that promotes a holistic attitude towards healing and formulates a community of sufferers (patients and caregivers) who identify with each other's personal experiences through the visually engaging memoirs. Furthermore, by exploring the recent global trends in graphic medicine, the chapter delineates how artists utilise online platforms to layer their narratives with audio-visual techniques and form communities of sufferers who actively share the author's experience through comment sections and kindred online facilities.

Chapter 2 provides a critical explanation for the use of Lakoff and Johnson's CMT theory by tracing the evolution of metaphor as a linguistic device to a phenomenon of lived experience. Deployed as a tool to conceptualise abstract emotions, the types and functions of visual metaphors in particular are explained in the chapter in the context of the CMT. Considering Sontag's criticism of metaphors of illness, the chapter discusses theorists like Frank, who deems metaphor not merely as a trope but as a significant figurative tool that assists in comprehending the diachronic and synchronic factors that affect one's illness experience. The chapter also espouses metaphors as an ideological tool by which biomedical claims of truth via objective standards are challenged and representation of multiple truths are validated.

Chapter 3 explores the question of representation, particularly visual representation, and its concomitant effects in socio-cultural spheres. Whereas every form of representation involves editions, simulations, additions, and deletions, the chapter delineates how these choices construct knowledge about the privileged and marginalised in the context of mental illness. Exploring the role of media in such knowledge construction, the chapter reviews sensationalised and distorted representations of the mentally ill in advertisements, movies, newspaper reports, and paintings. Taking cues from the theoretical postulates of Hall, Treichler, Edgar, Roth, and others, the chapter exposes prejudicial and discriminatory attitudes that are legitimised and normalised through social stigma. Apart from popular discourses, the chapter also examines statistics, medical definitions, and perspectives on mental illness, all of which tend to universalise the patient's experience through stock images and symptomatic diagnostic categories.

In response to the prevailing exclusionary patterns of representing mental illness, Chapter 4 proposes graphic memoirs as a counter-discourse to the extant stereotypical representations of mental illness that trivialise patient voices and perspectives. The chapter argues that personal accounts restore the language of mental illness, unlike popular and medical representations that follow patterns of exclusion. Accordingly, through contextualising graphic memoirs like *Marbles* and *Rx*, the chapter addresses the characterisation of distinct embodiment types through verbo-visual metaphors. It also explores the significance of the author's own visual narrative in renegotiating and renewing cultural and medical perceptions of these bodies/minds that have been distorted by popular media representations and biomedical prescriptions of mental disorders. Further, the chapter foregrounds the agency entailed in wielding control over self-image representation and deconstruction of the sanity/insanity binary. These theoretical concerns are addressed in this chapter by contextualising them in available bipolar disorder representation in movies, short films, and comics, and juxtaposing their major themes with bipolar disorder representations in graphic memoirs like *Marbles* and *Rx*. The chapter close-reads specific episodes from these memoirs to delineate how they utilise comics as a site of productive resistance against medical dogma and popular bipolar disorder stereotypes through subversion and ironic simulations. The chapter explicates the function of visual metaphors that performatively deconstruct the sanity/insanity binary and unsettle the fixity of such categorisations to challenge depersonalisation of the mentally ill.

Chapter 5 examines fictional OCD and schizophrenia narratives to delineate the creative potential of spatial and stylistic metaphors in picturing the patient's mental landscape. The metaphors deployed in these narratives on mental disorders, which are characterised by hallucinations and uncontrollable emotions, are significant, in that they seek to recreate the patient's subjective world, which is often deemed insignificant in clinical encounters. The chapter argues that an awareness of the patient's perspective, which is often suspended in the middle ground of triumphalism and fatalism, would facilitate relational identities, neutralise negative stereotypes, and dismantle debilitating clinical hierarchies. Moving beyond biomedical prescriptivism and claims to objectivity, the graphic narratives, *Swallow Me Whole* and *The Nao of Brown*, represent alternate realities as experienced by the patients themselves. Departing from clinical mental illness descriptions like schizophrenia, which label patients as unreasonable and without emotions, these narratives vividly manifest the complex and insightful nature of their life world.

The final core chapter explicates how metaphors are developed through conventional and creative ways to represent the experience of depression. By close-reading instances from several graphic memoirs on depression, including *Depresso, Psychiatric Tales*, and *Hyperbole and a Half*, the chapter proposes that while conventional metaphors that are drawn from the image bank of metaphors illustrate DEPRESSION IS DOWN/DEPRESSION IS FRAGMENTED conceptually, creative metaphors encapsulate the singular experience of depression through unique stylistic techniques and imaginative association with concrete conceptual categories. The chapter further discusses how these authors resort to stylistic techniques, emanatas, and novel conceptual associations to metaphorically convey the tacit experience of depression that is unavailable in medical discourse. Thereby, these graphic memoirists speak truth to power by owning their diagnosis through visual metaphors that offer ingress into the patient's lived reality.

The present study establishes the select graphic memoirs and narratives as vital intellectual sites for interrogating the contradictions and hierarchal power relations inherent in clinical and socio-cultural spheres that surround mental illness. This study suggests that these narratives attest to the critical necessity of reconfiguring popular perceptions on mental illness and cultural tendencies towards the mentally ill in the light of creative metaphors that encapsulate the trepidations caused by internal and social stigmas. Such subjective elucidations of patient's experience engender a parallel counter-discourse that stimulates a rethinking of mental illness as a singular experience that "create[s] a linguistic, co-created place for transactions and translations between patients [and] medical specialists" (Kristeva et al. 57) and the public. Problematising the politics of representation, this study theorises visual metaphors as counter-diagnostic tools that foster creative and novel representations of mental illness while critiquing biomedical models that attempt to normalise, homogenise, and pathologise mental conditions. Visualising the 'invisible' through the sufferer's own metaphorical expressions, these graphic memoirs transpire affective knowledge and posit meaningful remedies for the personal and socio-cultural quandaries of the mentally ill.

Though this study delineates multiple aspects of the illness experience, identity, and cultural influences within the rubric of conceptual metaphorical mappings, it is limited in expanding its contours towards cognitive/conceptual semantics, cognitive neuroscience, or cross-cultural cognition in relation to mental illness and metaphor creation. This study does not include primary sources from Japanese manga or Franco-Belgian *bandes dessinées* apropos of the specific issues that are faced by British and American authors/patients.

However, the present study does facilitate future research on mental illness, graphic memoirs, and visual metaphors in productive ways. Broadening the fields of cognitive linguistics and biomedicine, our observations could be effectively utilised in exploring the nature of metaphorical mappings and their impact on the human mind. Such a confluence of metaphorical and biomedical theories would unravel the effect of creative metaphorical mappings on recovery and healing. On the other hand, such research would also reveal complexities of narrative structures and visual metaphors that generate stock patterns and binaries that influence attitudes and perceptions towards the mentally ill. In essence, such studies would facilitate productive doctor-patient interactions and humanise mental illness to a greater extent through empirical means. Second, future studies on online mental illness narratives by patients/caregivers would expand the vistas of the current study to explore questions about online community formation via comments and sharing, audio-visual techniques that enhance the potential of comics, and the politics involved in the production and distribution of such webcomics through social media platforms.

## Reference List

Kristeva, Julia, et al. "Cultural Crossings of Care: An Appeal to the Medical Humanities." *Med Humanit*, vol. 44, 2018, pp. 55–58. doi: 10.1136/medhum-2017-011263.

# Index